Best Time To Eat & Exercise Guide

What the research tells us . . .

VINCE ROZIER

ISBN: 0991322444
ISBN-13: 978-0991322442
STEP ONE Publishing

DEDICATION

Who does not desire live a healthier life. Yes, there are those who, for some reason, have chosen not to make the effort. There are those who may not know how to and, thus, do not properly try. There are those who do not currently see the need and believe they will make a change when a doctor tells them it is necessary. Although, at this point, it is usually too late.

There are others who simply have given up. They have repeatedly made attempts to make a change for their lives and for the sake of their health. However, for some reason, that change was not enough. More information , effort, or some other element was needed to make a life lasting change.

This book is dedicated to these people. It is not expected that this book will be the magic pill to weight loss or a healthier life. However, it is hoped that the time spent with this book will allow the reader to get one step closer to the change that has been desired.

ACKNOWLEDGMENTS

Thank you to my friends and associates who took the time to research and contribute to this project. You are helping others to live the lives they desire to live with the health they seek to possess.

Medical Disclaimer

The author and researchers of the book are not medical doctors nor do they perform as ones on television. No one involved in the researching or writing of the materials in this book is an expert (or like the once popular commercial - stayed in a Holiday Inn the night prior to writing its materials).

The materials contained in this book are intended to provide helpful suggestions to allow the reader to live a healthier lifestyle. It is not intended to diagnose or treat any injury, disease, or illness. Additionally, this book is not be read or considered an alternative to a trained medical physician or other medical expert. The ideas offered within this book should not be considered as a means to cure or prevent any health problem or condition. Consult your physician prior to making any modifications to your dietary regiment, begin any new exercise program, or have any questions concerning matters contained in this book.

Those readers with particular conditions such as pregnancy, injury, disease, etc. should not make any modifications offered within this book without consulting a physician.

The author and publisher specifically disclaim all responsibility for any liability, loss, or risk, personal or otherwise, that is incurred as a consequence, directly or indirectly, from the use or application of any contents of this book. Whereas this book contains information regarding products from specific manufactures, always read product labels before using products. Moreover, the author and publisher are not responsible for claims made by manufacturers. The thoughts suggested in this book have not been reviewed by a physician, manufacturer, nor the US Food and Drug Administration.

CONTENTS

Introduction

So many people are obsessed with losing weight and there are countless strategies to choose from to reach your personal goals. From what to eat, to how much to eat, and what not to eat, there is always a new tweak for dieters to achieve better results.

In finding the diet that works for you, it is vital to think consider what habits you regularly incorporate into your lifestyle. During the process of modifying eating habits or cutting out different foods, an important fact must be remembered and not neglected - eating is a natural process of life. Moreover, going to extremes in an effort to lose weight can have terrible and unexpected consequences.

Throughout the remaining pages, you will find information to help you to create a personal diet that will specifically work for you. Yes, a one size fits all diet may have proven results in the short term, but it may not serve your permanent lifestyle. Here, you will find information that is set to give you discretion in choosing what you eat and help you understand the impact of your choices.

1

Metabolism by the clock

Optimize Meal Timing For Success

Your right! A vital step in dieting for weight loss is knowing what foods to eat. However, simply knowing what foods to eat may not be enough to get the results you want. Knowing when to eat is also a key and important factor in keeping weight and health management.

Just like we may become accustomed to going to sleep and waking up at certain times, our bodies may also learn when to expect food. Training your body when to expect food makes it better at processing it. Your body can then follow that schedule in order to naturally achieve the best results.

For those who have taken the time to research and read dieting books, many answers may seem obvious. Yet, with all the diets that have been promoted, it can be difficult to discern which diet to follow. From South Beach to Akins, from low carbs to no carbs, what and when to eat may eventually become confusing.

Should carbs be consumed at dinner?

Can I be healthy without eating any carbs at all?

Will drinking cold water after a meal be damaging to my digestive system?

Will eating fruit after meat cause a nutrient deficiency?

With all the information that is available to help establish a healthy lifestyle, using the clock is the one constant that will always provide clear direction. However, it is still important to understand some essential facts about a clock-guided, healthy lifestyle.

For instance, there is no time of day that eating junk food is beneficial for you. On the other hand, there may be a time when its negative impact can be reduced. Likewise, there is no time strategy to correctly consider carrot cake a vegetable. There may, however, be a time to include vegetables in your daily diet. Whether eating the healthiest food or drinking wine to reduce cholesterol, knowing the right time as a part of your lifestyle can make the difference between something being a detriment or benefit to your health.

Breakfast - The Metabolism Power Meal

There are no secret foods like the cartoon character Popeye the sailor eating a can of spinach. Eating breakfast as the largest meal, however, allows for ample time during the day for those calories to be burned off naturally, even without exercise. All the day's activities at work and the movements used during your daily routines become burners for the calories consumed at breakfast. (Otherwise, when dinner is the biggest meal, the body is trying to catch up from the night before.) Then when exercise during the day is added in, the benefits can be even greater!

* *

<u>BBB</u>

"A <u>Bigger</u> <u>Breakfast</u> is <u>Better</u>."

As the saying goes, "Eat breakfast like a king, lunch like a prince, and dinner like a pauper."

* *

Some diets may encourage fasting or skipping

4

meals as a part of weight loss. However, most people will find it difficult to live a lifestyle in which you have to know what day of the week it is to determine whether to eat or not. Following the 3 B's lifestyle will serve as a guide during a busy work week, on vacation, or enjoying a relaxing day at home.

Going Against The Norm With Dinner

Culturally, many people reserve their largest meal of the day for dinner. This indeed is sometimes an event or a positive time for families to gather together at the end of the day. Dinner is often used as a time for friends to gather. Also, dinner may be a time when it is finally possible to relax with a favorite dish after a long and stressful day.

Waiting until the end of the day for the largest meal, however, leaves very little time for the calories consumed to be burned off naturally. There typically is not much time left over for exercise after one's food has been digested. Instead, most people do the opposite of what is beneficial for weight loss.

Most people find themselves eating dinner and then doing little that is active for the remainder of the day. This is amplified by the simple act of watching television while eating. This only encourages us to continue eating until the program is over, even though we would have stopped after 15 minutes at a dinner table.

Whether it watching television, connecting with others on the computer, reading, or just sleeping, many common post dinner activities require being sedentary. The result is that someone may have done a great job of total calorie consumption throughout the day, but counteract all of their hard work at the end. Thus, they still end up gaining weight by eating a large dinner. So, why not flip the menu!

Instead of making dinner the biggest meal of the day, try making breakfast the largest meal of the day. With a proper, large breakfast, there is even less of a desire for snacking on junky treats during the day. Then, eating healthy snacks create the sensation of simply topping of where someone has already been filled up with the first meal of the day.

* *

Quick Tip

There should be at least 2-3 hours between bedtime and the last meal of the day. Eating too close to sleeping at night has been associated with a variety of problems such as strokes, insomnia, sleep apnea, acid reflux and weight gain.

* *

Poor Meal Timing - Skipping Meals

In the process of trying to improve one's health, some people are convinced that drastic changes are necessary to achieve the desired results. This may be true if someone is extremely unhealthy in their diet. Nevertheless, taking drastic measures in dieting can certainly backfire.

Some strategies suggest skipping meals and eating only a particular group of nutrients while ignoring others. Unfortunately, a lot of people follow advice from the wrong sources, implement poor dieting tips, and become frustrated when they do not see the desired results. The human body is a complex creation that requires numerous and varied "building blocks" in order to function properly.

There is no sense in depriving the body of what it naturally needs. That type of deprivation is a plan for guaranteed crashes, fatigue, and potential illness. Meanwhile, a good, balanced eating lifestyle will include sets of meals that should have a little of everything - proteins, carbohydrates, and yes, even some fats.

At first, it seems like a brilliantly simple, yet efficient idea - skip a meal, skip some calories. Yet, that is not the whole picture. Skipping meals triggers a hardwired response in the human body. The body interprets the lack of food to mean that no other food will be received anytime soon. Therefore, the body functions to process food more slowly. In other words, ones metabolism is slowed by this food deprivation.

As a result, the body spends less energy and retains more calories as it awaits the next meal. Instead of losing weight, the body begins to slowly gain weight. For most people who regularly skip meals, this could not be further from their original goal! This, therefore, leads to a logical conclusion. Eating more (yet smaller meals) can be beneficial in the arena of weight loss.

By eating smaller meals, the metabolic rate may remain actually speed up, without consuming more calories from larger meals. There are even more benefits to this way of eating, which will be discussed later. *However, knowing the right time to eat these smaller meals is key.*

Some people choose to utilize the strategy of intermittent fasting. Here, the goal is to lose weight by tricking the body into missing an occasional meal, without the unintended consequence of slowing down the metabolism. This has been found to have its benefits if used one to two times per week. However, caution must be implemented to make sure that binge eating does not occur after fasting to make up for the meals missed. Also, attention and careful thought must go into this planning to keep tract of the days.

The Science of Meal Timing

One of the primary reasons for having several smaller meals is based around the human body's metabolism. Metabolism is basically the way food is processed into energy. For some people, it is fast. For others, it is slower or even faster. A May 2005 study in the American Journal of Clinical Nutrition has determined that frequent meals are a crucial factor in keeping the metabolic rate high.

While it is true that the speed at which someone metabolizes food can be hereditary, the metabolic rate (the rate at which energy is generated and spent) depends largely on lifestyle choices. Other factors include age, gender, and specific illnesses. For example, thyroid gland problems may be responsible for a 3 percent increase or decrease in someone's metabolic rate. (Those who are concerned about their metabolic rate being unusually low/ slow, may find it valuable to consult a doctor.)

In addition to metabolism benefits, small, frequent meals also play a part in balancing blood sugar. Blood sugar is exactly what it sounds like - the measureable amount of sugar or glucose present in the blood. Having multiple small meals helps to stabilize and maintain proper blood sugar levels and helps a person avoid sugar cravings, which are common factors in weight gain.

Our brains require enormous amounts of sugar to

work properly. Genevieve Sherrow, a professor of the Department of Nutrition and Exercise Science in Bastyr University, states that a lack of glucose typically causes headaches, fatigue, anxiety or even depression. On the other hand, a surplus of sugar may lead to diabetes and other complications.

* *

Quick Tip from Sumo Wrestlers

In order to maintain their curved figure (one large continuous curve that makes them so round like a big "O"), sumo wrestlers:

1. NEVER eat breakfast

2. ONLY eat 1-2 meals a day

3. Sleep after eating

4. Drink large amounts of beer

Do not skip meals for your diet unless you are working to become a sumo wrestler!

* *

Snacks

Snacking on the wrong foods may also be extremely tempting when dealing with those nasty sugar cravings. It is important, however, to consider that the sensations of hunger and the binge eating that naturally follows from prolonged hunger are something one should try to avoid. Through a healthy diet and proper eating habits, hunger can easily be minimized. All it takes is the addition regularly eating the right snacks and proper hydration. Just remember, a snack is fine. Making it another meal will only cause you to gain weight!

Metabolism with Eating and Exercise

It is widely understood that exercise combined with a proper diet provides the healthiest way to lose weight, gain muscle mass, or attain overall improved fitness. It is also true that the right foods must be paired with the right exercise to get the right results. For example some diets are considered healthy and low in calories. These diets, however, may not be best for those who indulge in very extensive strength and cardio workouts. This is because these workouts require increased amounts of energy.

To lose weight while trying to eat the right foods with exercise, it is important to understand what is considered ones metabolic window. The metabolic window is a 30-45-minute period following strength exercising during which your body shifts from breaking down body tissues (catabolic state) and organs to building them up (anabolic state).

After exercise, taking advantage of the 30-45 minute metabolic window right after a workout is vital to attaining desired results. By understanding the metabolic window and making the right choice about when and what to eat, you can lose fat and replace any proteins lost. Meanwhile, eating the right carbohydrates and proteins at the right time can help you lose weight and build muscle at the same time.

Another key component to the metabolic window is the Glycemic Index and Glycemic Load. Understanding Glycemic Index (GI) and Glycemic Load (GL) can also serve as a key in the effort to learn what foods may provide fuel for a workout and stabilize the body afterwards. These models provide information about the amount of glucose contained in different foods.

For example, the body uses glucose for a short time at the beginning of high intensity exercises. Endurance exercises (those that typically last for more than 45 minutes) deplete glycogen stores. The body must then rely on the breakdown of fat and protein that is stored in the body to provide energy. (*The discussion of Glycemic Index and Load will follow in the chapter on Carbohydrates.*)

This process of burning through glycogen to get to fat and protein is good for those who want to lose fat. However, it may serve as a double-edged sword for those seeking to bulk up with muscle. If done regularly, it may also lead to some loss of lean muscle mass. Those seeking to add muscle mass should consider this because the body burns energy to recuperate and repair muscles even after exercise stops.

During recovery period after exercise, one can take medium or even high GI foods, especially carbohydrates and proteins, to stimulate protein synthesis and glycogen storage. Because people exercise at different times of the day, it is not possible to design one strict schedule for everyone. Whether you go to the gym in the morning, afternoon or evening, it is important remember the metabolic window. Take advantage of the right foods during this 30-45 minutes after you work out and take greater control of your weight.

Prepare Your Metabolism

Properly timed meals should also help alleviate the distracting sensation of hunger. This balance will improve both your physical and psychological state. One of the most important benefits of becoming accustomed to eating on a schedule is the avoidance of troublesome eating habits, like binge eating. **If a tasty dessert is not on the schedule, it may be hard to fit it in!**

It is important to note that while exercise is important in becoming fit and healthy, it is not everything. No amount of exercise can be efficient enough to compensate for an unhealthy diet or poor eating habits. Over the course of time, eating healthy is not about making up for one day. It is about a lifetime of health. So, seek to incorporate all of these methods in order to get better results, and maintain a good looking, healthy body.

2

Timing exercise

for your lifestyle

Exercise has been shown to have countless and obvious positive health effects: weight loss, improved strength and endurance, greater mental focus, stress release, reduced chances of getting various diseases, etc. Researchers are now going further than just detailing the fact that exercise is beneficial to one's overall health. They are now examining whether the time of day affects the quality of a workout and its overall benefits.

Does it matter when you do certain exercises?

As with many things in life, the quick answer is, "It depends." A more specific answer is, "It depends on what you want." As studies continue to be done, experts are concluding that certain exercises, done at certain periods of the day, may result in maximum performance and effectiveness. Meanwhile, the same exercises done at different times of the day may not always produce the same optimal performance. Additionally, performing certain exercises at times that do not allow for peak performance may still lead to other positive results. Timing exercise may serve as an effective way of increasing your metabolic rate, burning additional calories, and even training for future events or performances.

The bottom line is that even though research is still new and ongoing, current evidence points to the fact that the time of day does indeed affect the quality of a workout. Now, let's look at the pros and cons of exercising at different times of the day and consider which exercises may work for you.

Morning

The highest percentage of people exercise in the morning. This is evident in the number of people at gyms, pools, yoga studios and the joggers running through neighborhoods at the break of dawn. Also, don't forget those who exercise to videos as a part of their morning ritual. The tendency for people to engage in these early morning adventures may be for several reasons.

For some, the morning is the best time simply because they have control of their schedule more than any other time of the day. Meanwhile, others feel that they are just not morning people and enjoy being able to ease into the day. They prefer a vigorous afternoon or evening workout.

The time that people choose to workout is often a personal choice that may not be related to health benefits at all. All are reasons that many choose to or not to begin the day with an easy or vigorous workout. So, let's take a look at the health related pros and cons of doing so.

Pros of morning exercise

• **You can burn more fat during a morning workout.**

Research from Northumbria University found that exercising in the morning on an empty stomach can burn up to 20% more body fat than exercising later in the day. While results may vary from person to person, this is because your body is low on glycogen first in the morning after having fasted during sleep. Glycogen, which is the form in which the body stores glucose, is burned with fat during exercise. Thus, when the glycogen level in the body is lower than after eating, the body can efficiently go to burning more fat.

• **It boosts your metabolism and ensures that it stays up all day long.**

Calories are not only burned during exercise. Calories are also burned during the recovery from the exercise that has already taken place. For instance, the process of rebuilding muscle after exercise requires energy. This rebuilding process is also a calorie burner. (This is especially true with weight lifting as the body repairs muscles torn and exercised during the process of lifting weights.) As a result, exercise performed first thing in the morning allows for more calories to be burned throughout the day. This rate at which calories are burned throughout the day may also increase with more intense morning workouts.

• **Better sleep at night.**

In a study carried out by Appalachian State University, individuals who woke up to exercise at 7:00 am were observed to sleep better and more deeply at night. Thus, being active first thing in the morning puts the body in a rhythm to rest and repeat the next day's exercise and activities.

• **Lowering of blood pressure.**

The same Appalachian State University study also indicated that the early morning exercisers experienced a 10 percent decrease in blood pressure throughout the day. At night, the blood pressure dropped by 25 percent.

• It makes one become more alert.

There may initially be a sluggishness to overcome with morning exercise. It may take some time before the stillness of night converts into the activeness required for exercise. Yet, when it does happen, the body becomes more alert and active. This alertness is maintained for hours into the day and can help improve work productivity.

In addition to lowering blood pressure and burning fat more efficiently, morning exercise is primarily beneficial for the stimulation it offers. The increased metabolism, alertness, and endorphin production ensures that your day starts off energized.

• You are more likely to be consistent with your workouts if you choose the morning period since there are not as many distractions.

Some people choose to exercise first thing in the morning because it is the time that they can most easily and consistently schedule their workout in the midst of a busy schedule. Some find that working out in the morning and showering at the gym, pool, or yoga studio makes sense and fits their schedule perfectly. Others find that they are able to maintain their fitness and weight if they run on the treadmill at home or through the neighborhood before the kids are awake.

Cons of morning exercise

• **Energy levels in the body are low in the morning.**

The transition from being asleep to being fully active may take longer depending on how rested someone feels. Not getting enough sleep the night before may make it difficult to find the energy the next morning. This may prevent one from engaging in high intensity exercise early in the morning.

• **Because muscles are still cold and stiff, there is an increase in the risk of injury.**

If there is only a limited amount of time for exercise, it may take some time for the body to loosen and become ready for an intense workout. If the muscles have not been warmed up, there is an increased chance of injury.

• **There is a danger of your muscle mass being burned together with fat due to low glycogen levels.**

It may seem to be a benefit to many people to burn additional calories and glucose with morning workouts. However, for those who are looking to maintain muscle, this may not be desired. This is particularly true if you exercise before taking breakfast.

Still, those who are looking to become chiseled and to have beach bodies should remember that no matter how big a muscle is, it cannot be seen if there is too much fat covering all the hard work that has been done. This is particularly important for those seeking to reveal a chiseled six pack.

• **For those who are not morning people, exercising in the morning everyday can be very challenging. It will require discipline and commitment to maintain a regular exercise schedule.**

Just knowing that you do not want to be up early in the morning may make you prefer to not workout at all if it means being up early in the day. The only morning exercise that is desired is to hit the snooze on the alarm.

Afternoon

In the afternoon, our body temperatures are higher and our muscles are no longer stiff and cold. It may also be the best time to get in a walk to find 30 minutes of silence.

Pros of afternoon exercise

• Less risk of injuries.

After getting into the regular flow of the day, the muscles have loosened and are no longer stiff. The extra amount of time to loosen the muscles and move into becoming active, therefore, is not required. Without this stiffness that comes with early exercising, muscles like hamstrings (that may result in injury if there is tightness during exercise) have become more flexible and allow for performance without the same risk of injury.

• Improved workout performance due to higher body temperature.

With increased body temperature and greater muscle fluidity, it becomes possible to have a more effective workout. Your muscles are stronger. So, you can better perform higher intensity exercises. Those same high intensity exercises may be difficult to energetically perform while fighting the drowsiness of sleep. They are now easier to complete once the afternoon arrives.

• It can help to get rid of the stress accumulated in the course of the day.

Once the day has begun to flow, the stressors of life begin to present themselves. Having the opportunity to exercise with deep breathing, increase blood flow, and a momentary break away from work or home can help to calm the body's response to stress. It is true that exercise may increase the release of cortisol, the hormone released by the adrenal gland as a response to stress. However, regular exercise allows for this release to be decreased by exercise. Thus, exercise during the afternoon only further assists in the process of becoming mentally relaxed in the midst of the day's stress.

• For some people, sticking to an afternoon routine is easy.

Not all schedules are created equal. The afternoon workout may be the best time of the day to maintain consistency in exercise for some but not for others. For some, morning child duties and school drop off may be the cause of getting to work early. This may, however, present the opportunity to have more time for lunch to exercise.

• Muscle repair function is at its best which improves exercise performance.

Cons of afternoon exercise

• The number of distractions in the afternoon means that most people will find it hard to maintain exercising consistency for many days.

These distractions can also limit the set exercise time. A busy morning may lead to a shorter exercise time in the afternoon.

• **Lung function is not at its best.**

This may affect breathing and lower the quality of any aerobic exercises. If you are exercising outside, there is more pollen, car exhaust, and dust that have accumulated, which can negatively affect your breathing.

Evening

A number of individuals prefer to exercise in the evening. Studies have shown that at around 6 o'clock in the evening, body temperature, hormones and lung function are at their peak. Indeed, it is a common occurrence to see gyms filled with people in the evening after work who are seeking to make it to a class, find a machine, or settle onto a weight lifting bench.

Pros of evening exercise

• **Peak body temperature allows for higher exercise performance especially, for those who plan on carrying out intense cardio exercises.**

• **Muscles are warm and the mind is alert, thus**

reducing the risk of injury.

• Fewer scheduled distractions for the rest of the day can help increase exercise time and quality.

• Evening workouts are great for reducing the stress accumulated during the day.

• As long as the exercise is not done within 2 hours of bedtime, it can help m facilitate better sleeping at night.

Cons of evening exercise

• There is not the same benefit of increased metabolism hours after exercising like there is in after exercising earlier in the day.

Once you begin to sleep, the body's metabolism drops. As a result, your body will not burn as many calories after you have completed your workout - unlike in the morning. Yes, the body will still receive some fat burning benefits from repairing muscles damaged during exercise. However, this will not be at the same rate as when exercise was performed in the morning.

• If the exercise time is too close to bedtime, it may interfere with a good night's sleep.

This is because one may get too energized from exercising, which in turn can prevent good sleep.

More intense exercises also cause the body's core temperature to increase, which may prevent sleep until the body has naturally cooled.

Best exercises for the time of day

Morning

Due to the low energy levels and muscle stiffness, go with low-intensity workouts for a warm up. Swimming, yoga, or even a 15 minute walk are some of the best exercises for morning to get the day going. Running is an exercise that is common for many in the morning. If this is the morning exercise, it is good to allow for some low intensity exercise to warm up the muscles. *Trying to warm up muscles with cold stretching, however, is not good and may result in injury.*

Most endurance events such as triathlons and marathons are often held in the morning. With these, it is good to engage in some movement to warm up the muscles prior to beginning.

Lunch/ Afternoon

This is the time of the day to get the best results in demanding exercises such as weight lifting, running and other cardio routines. There is still some freshness from the morning, but there is also the increase of body temperature and greater flexibility to reduce the likelihood of injury.

Evening

The evening is best for high intensity workouts. This is the best period of the day to work on building muscle density. Exercises such as weight lifting are, therefore, recommended.

* *

Quick Tip

Consistency and persistence should be your priorities.

Set a certain period for exercise and stick with that period.

* *

Best time for you

Ultimately, the best period to workout will depend on a number of factors such as your schedule, goals, and lifestyle. Some thought to help you find what works best for you are:

If you plan on burning fat fast, capitalize on morning exercise on an empty stomach.

If you want to build your muscles, avoid exercising in the morning and do it in the afternoon or in the evening.

If you have a job that allows for a regularly scheduled lunch, your lunch break could be a good time to hit a nearby gym before heading back to the office. This is particularly true if you find yourself working late nights that make it difficult to get up early in the morning.

If you are crunched for time at home and simply want to get complete some level activity, consider walking during lunch or after work before going home.

3

Carbohydrates as sugar?

What are carbs?

In recent years, few classifications of food have received as much attention in the dieting community as have carbohydrates. Some argue that the way to lose weight is to avoid any and all carbohydrates. Others contend that the way to have energy for exercise is to load on carbohydrates before exercise. So, what are carbs and what do they do?

Carbohydrates (carbs) are a class of food that provides energy to the body, brain, and nervous system. During digestion, carbohydrates cause the body to produce glucose (sugar), which is then converted into energy to support bodily functions and physical activity.

Carbohydrates initiate the body's production of glucose similar to the way the body responds to sugar. The body uses glucose immediately or stores it in the body for when it is needed. Whether dieting or not, most people understand that a steady consumption of sugar will not produce weight loss. Therefore, most people who want to lose weight will want to avoid those foods that cause the body to act as though it is ingesting sugar.

However, all foods which contain carbohydrates or that are considered carbohydrates do not fall into the category of bad foods. In fact, there are different categories of carbohydrates. There are simple (sugary) carbohydrates and complex (starches) carbohydrates. *(Foods containing fiber are often considered carbohydrates also. However, the topic of fibers will be discussed later.)* All of which may cause the body to respond in completely different ways.

In order to know when to eat carbohydrates, it is important to first understand which type of carbohydrate is being consumed.

Simple Carbohydrates

Foods containing simple carbohydrates do not have a detailed or complicated chemical structure. They are constructed with one or two chains of sugar and typically do not have a significant nutritional value. Because of their simple structure, simple carbohydrates are foods that are rapidly digested by the body. The simple structure of these carbs allows them to provide a quick source of energy.

This fast-paced, digesting process is why simple carbs have been considered by some as good sources of energy during endurance exercises. Whatever is consumed can be quickly converted in a manner similar to a sugar spike. However, if simple carbohydrates are not burned off or used for energy during a workout, all is left over and not used will be stored as fat.

Additionally, the fast processing of simple carbohydrates can quickly impact blood sugar levels. This immediate reaction negatively increases and spikes blood sugar levels. It can be a danger to those who are diabetic. Thus, those who are diabetic should be cautious when consuming simple carbohydrates.

Simple carbs provide extra calories. As such, consumption of larger quantities may be related to weight gain.

Examples of simple carbs are:

White flour	Chips
Candy	Doughnuts
Fruit juice	Cookies
Cereals	Cake
Soda	White rice
Table sugar	White bread
French Fries	Crackers

Processed foods that contain simple carbohydrates often include the following as ingredients:

Brown sugar

Corn sweetener

Corn syrup

Dextrose

Fructose

Fruit juice concentrates

Glucose

High-fructose corn syrup

Honey

Invert sugar

Lactose

Maltose

Malt Syrup

Molasses

Raw sugar

Sucrose

Sugar

Syrup

Complex Carbohydrates

Complex carbohydrates possess a more detailed chemical structure and are constructed with several chains of molecules. This more complex structure requires a longer process to break down and digest the complex carbohydrates. Along with a longer digesting process, the impact on blood sugar is more gradual because the glucose that is created is not immediately introduced into the blood stream. Thus, there is not as much caution required by diabetics in consuming complex carbohydrates.

Contained in the detailed structure of complex carbohydrates is a more nutritious value than that of simple carbohydrates. So, consumption of complex carbohydrates are not always considered a source of empty, weight-gaining calories. Some carbs that are considered complex also contain a significant amount of fiber, which can be helpful during digestion as well.

Like simple carbohydrates, complex carbs also serve as energy producers. The energy produced by complex carbs, however, is not always quickly burned off. This may depend on the source and purity of the carbohydrate. For example, some foods may be processed or contain additives that have resulted in natural complex carbohydrates being diminished of their full nutritional value.

* *

Quick Tip

Get in the habit of reading the ingredients listed on packaged foods. If you see enriched wheat flour, sugar, or corn syrup, then recognize that the product contains refined carbohydrates, which are all bad for health. The best way to avoid enriched carbohydrates is to buy products in their unprocessed, wholesome form. Avoid bread, pasta, cookies, and crackers as they are normally cooked with enriched flour.

* *

Examples of complex carbohydrates are:

Asparagus	Dill Pickles	Plums
Bagel	Dried apricots	Porridge
Baked beans	Eggplant	Oats
Bananas	Garbanzo beans	Prunes
Beans	Granary Bread	Soybeans
Broccoli	Grapefruits	Spaghetti
Brown bread	Kidney beans	Spinach
Brown rice	Legumes	Split peas
Brussels	Lentils	Sprouts
Sprouts	Lettuce	Strawberries
Buckwheat	Multi-grain	Sweet potato
bread	bread	Tomatoes
Cabbage	Navy beans	Turnip Greens
Carrots	Oatmeal	Watercress
Cassava	Okra	Whole Barley
Cauliflower	Onions Oranges	Whole grain
Celery	Root vegetables	Wild rice
Chickpeas	Peas	Yam
Cucumbers	Pinto beans	Zucchini

Whole grains versus Whole wheat

The difference between whole grains and whole wheat is that whole grain still possesses the entire kernel of the grain; the grain, germ, and endosperm are all intact. Conversely, whole wheat has to go through a refining process that removes the bran and the germ, only the endosperm is left. When the grain goes through a process in which it may be cracked, crushed, or flaked (as may be the case with flakes or cereal), the grain must maintain a similar amount of bran, germ, and endosperm to still be considered whole grain. Once the grains are refined or enriched, the natural qualities originally present have been modified and diminished.

Unfortunately, whole wheat has most of the nutritional content removed since the majority of fiber and vitamins are in the wheat germ and wheat bran that are shed during the refining process. While it's difficult to tell the difference between the two, whole grain has a richer taste and dense texture than whole wheat. The only way to be sure of knowing is to read the package label.

Breakfast Carbs (Good & Bad)

There is a reason that breakfast is described as the most important meal of the day. You have fasted all night. Your body needs fuel for the day. The body's glucose levels are sensitive and need to be balanced for the coming day. Thus, it is very important to take note of what you eat during the morning. Eating the right foods that are rich in the right carbohydrates can provide your body with the energy it needs for the day.

If you choose to eat carbs for breakfast, eating good complex carbohydrates in the morning will provide your body with energy to set you on the right path for the whole day. Since complex carbohydrates take longer to breakdown, you will have a full-stomach feeling that will help to avoid overeating. Some of the foods you can consider for healthy carbohydrates in the morning include oatmeal, berries, whole wheat grain, fruits, milk, cereal etc.

However, eating a butter saturated grain or wheat muffin that contains berries in the middle of sugary, enriched flour

a) does not make it a good or healthy alternative
b) will not help maintain blood sugar levels and
c) will not provide a long lasting feeling of satiety (being full).

i. Avoid Early Morning Sugary Carbs

In the morning, your body is burning fat that was stored during the night in order to provide your body with fuel in the morning. Because sugar is easily digested and absorbed in the blood stream, eating sugary carbohydrates in the morning will lead to increased glucose levels. Increased glucose levels in the blood leads to the release of insulin. This changes the body from burning fat to storing it. So, even exercising in the morning will not provide the best benefits because the sugar is being burned as fuel and not the body's fat. This is one of the reasons people exercise but never see any changes in their weight.

Avoid bad carbohydrates in the morning like white bread, cakes, juice, muffins, etc. Bad carbohydrates add unhealthy sugars into the body and may make you feel fatigued for the whole day, all because of what you had for breakfast. In the long term, they contribute to weight gain and promote heart disease and diabetes.

ii. Whole grains in morning

Whole grain foods are low in saturated fats. This helps lower cholesterol levels and avoid serious diseases such as heart disease and diabetes. Eating whole grains with fat in the morning will provide your body with good fats that will provide energy for the whole day. It will also help fight bad fats and cholesterol that will contribute to overall better health. An example of whole grain with fats is a bowl of yogurt with added grains.

Avoid Late Night Carbohydrates

Avoid carbohydrates late at night or before you go to bed. We have discussed that carbohydrates are used by the body as energy or stored for future use. The spike caused by carbs will provide more energy at night that may make it difficult to sleep through the night.

Even if you find that you are able to sleep throughout the night after eating carbs, there will be no time to burn off what has been consumed. Much of the sugar will be stored as fat. Again, there is an increased chance of having elevated sugar levels. Eating within an hour of bed has also been related to an increased rate of strokes.

Carbohydrates When Exercising

3- 4 hours before workouts

Consuming carbohydrates 3-4 hours before exercise may serve as a source for sustained energy to prevent muscle loss. This amount of time between eating and exercising may allow you to use the carbohydrates as energy and to replenish depleted glycogen from the exercise. Although there may not be a truly beneficial time to consume simple carbohydrates, this may be the time that may allow for them to be burned off quickly.

During endurance workouts

Many long distance athletes who compete in activities such as marathons and triathlons become programmed to consume gels, gu, beans, or other forms of simple carbs at specific times during their events. Meanwhile, a number of endurance athletes are now beginning to follow low carbohydrate diets. They have learned that a training with a diet that that allows them to burn fat as fuel is better and more consistent than relying on carbs and glucose. Nevertheless, consuming simple carbs during endurance events is still widely utilized as a source of fuel for those who regularly consume carbohydrates.

There are now other non-sugary alternatives available for endurance athletes. For example, in 2014, 38 year old Meb Keflezighi used the non-sugary product, Generation UCan, to fuel him to victory in the Boston Marathon instead of using a traditional sugary gu or gel.

Post work out

After working out, your body has used a significant amount of energy and needs to be replenished.

When following a diet that does include carbohydrates, eating healthy carbohydrates after working out is be beneficial. The consumption of complex carbs after working out will help the body become more accustomed to breaking down these carbs and using them for fuel.

Carb Diet Options

There are many diet options to choose from to help you consume the right amount of carbohydrates. Some of the diets include:

Atkins diet

This is a low carb high protein diet. The diet encourages people to cut out carbs for rapid weight loss.

Low carbs

The low carb diet does allow for consuming a limited amount of some complex carbohydrates. The source of complex carbohydrates on the low carb diet should be from foods that are not processed.

No sugar no grains (NSNG)

This is a high protein diet that restricts sugar and carb intake in your diet. NSNG directs that dieters consume foods high in protein to maintain lean muscle tissue for enhanced metabolism. As a result, the body is conditioned to burn fat more efficiently.

Choose Your Own Path

It is important to take note of the carbs you consume. *Like calories, not all carbs are the same.* To be on the safe side, always read the ingredients on food packages and make a conscious decision to eat healthily.

* *

Quick Tip

If you cannot understand or pronounce all of the ingredients contained in your food, choose something else.

* *

It is becoming increasingly accepted that some carbohydrates are useful in a diet, but only those that have specific nutritional value. Fruits and vegetables that contain carbohydrates may be appropriate when trying to avoid carbohydrates. However, avoiding carbohydrates found in grains may lead to positive changes in a diet.

More nutritionists, doctors, and athletes are joining the no grains/ no sugars bandwagon. This may be hard for some to accept. It may be difficult to convert from a turkey sandwich to just turkey. However, the positive results will not be hard to receive.

Ultimately, you will have to find the right balance that works for you. Find the right balance, and learn to time it right for the best results.

4

Understanding Blood Sugar

In discussing carbohydrates, fruits, and other foods that contain glucose, it is important to discuss how glucose impacts blood sugar. Typically, the glucose levels in your blood rise after eating any kind of food. Utilizing Glycemic Index (GI) and Glycemic Load (GL) serve as guides to understanding the relationship between food and blood sugar.

Glycemic Index

The Glycemic Index allows for measuring the impact that certain carbohydrates will have on blood sugar. The Glycemic Index assists in understanding how quickly glucose levels rise after eating certain types of food. So, instead of only measuring the amount of carbohydrates or calories in a meal, someone may choose to give attention to how a particular food rates on the Glycemic Index.

For each type of food on the GI, a figure is given as a percentage of 100 percent glucose. The Glycemic

Index seeks to give an estimate of how much each unit gram of available carbohydrate in a particular food type increases your glucose level.

Based on the Glycemic Index, foods can fall into either of three categories:

1) Low GI ,

2) Medium GI, and

3) High GI.

Foods with a low GI may better satisfy someone at a meal without causing blood sugar levels to spike. Meanwhile, foods that have a higher GI initiate the release of more insulin into the blood and account for the higher amounts of sugar that will be present in the body. This insulin allows for the sugar to be converted and utilized for energy. With increased levels of sugar and insulin being used for energy, there is no longer the need to burn stored fat. *Thus, while foods with a high GI may not be high in caloric content, they may prevent weight loss by only burning sugar and not allowing fat to be burned.*

There are now a number of health concerns known to be related to the regular consumption of higher GI foods. Hypertension, diabetes, and heart disease have been linked with regularly having high insulin levels. Meanwhile, regular consumption of low GI foods (and thus lower insulin levels) are now associated with decreased risk of cardiovascular disease, type 2 diabetes, depression, and certain cancers.

Glycemic Load

Knowing the GI of a food may give rise to the consideration that someone would be able to have a large meal full of foods with a low GI. One of the limitations of the Glycemic Index is that it does not take into account the amount of available carbohydrate eaten per serving. To provide accuracy on how certain foods will impact the body on a per serving basis, another measure known as Glycemic Load (GL) was created. Like the Glycemic Index, a GL level may fall into any of three categories: low GL (less than 10), medium GL (11-19) and high GL (greater than 20).

Both GI and GL affect caloric intake as well as exercise and therefore weight management. Foods with low to medium GI usually have low GL and contain low calories.

To learn the Glycemic Index/ Load of your favorite foods, see the Appendix.

* *

Endurance Athletes

If someone is concerned about maintaining blood sugar levels or having enough energy to burn during an endurance event, low GI foods may initially provide concern. This concern may depend on what their body has become accustomed to during endurance training. For example, if they have trained with a plan to burn foods or substances that are sugary or high on the Glycemic Index, it may be difficult to quickly transition into a new fueling strategy during a race. However, many endurance athletes are now learning to use fat as fuel instead of relying on the glucose from carbohydrates. In doing such, they avoid blood sugar spikes that go along with carbohydrate fueling.

* *

5

Fruits (too sugary?)

Eating fruits is, without a doubt, important to our health and well-being. We have grown accustomed to considering fruits to be amongst the best types of foods we can eat. No matter the fruit, they are widely believed to be healthy and pure regardless of when they are consumed. However, to avail the many benefits that fruits have to offer, one must incorporate the right fruits into their diet the proper way and at the right time.

Preparation and storage

One of the great aspects of fruit is the ease required in preparing them for consumption. Usually, a simple rinse or washing is all that is required. They can easily be packaged and then later consumed. As with anything, what is fresh is better. Fresh fruits have the benefit of containing a higher percentage of nutrients.

Some may find it appropriate to use fruits that have been stored in a can or that have been dried as a helpful means for storing their fruit. Canned or dried fruits may seem to be better than none. However, this is not always the case.

Be aware that certain preservatives are added to canned fruits to make sure that the fruit can be maintained in a form other than its natural condition. Some preservatives such as salt, increased sugars, or forms of sugar like fructose and corn syrup are often added to the fruit's natural sweetness. This takes away from the potentially great benefits the fruit can provide in its natural state and may actually add negative effects. So, it may be better to avoid canned or dried fruit, depending on what has been added.

Eating Fruits On An Empty Stomach

In examining when the best time of day to consume fruits is, let us first consider how to eat fruits. The how of eating fruits is whether it is better to eat them on an empty stomach or if the same benefits can be received after eating other foods. While there are proven benefits to eating fruits before certain types of food, there have also been varied beliefs and unsubstantiated theories about the consequences of eating fruit after or during a meal with other foods.

For a period of time, some diets proposed that fruits needed to be eaten before meals (morning before breakfast, noon before lunch and evening just before dinner) to get the most out of them. The thought was that eating fruit at the beginning of a meal increased the efficiency of absorbing the fruit's nutrients into the body. The logic followed that when fruits are eaten with (or after) a meal, the foods mix. Then, the stomach cannot receive or sort out all that has been introduced into the digestive system. The result would be the rotting of fruit atop of other foods in the stomach.

In fact, this theory suggests that specific types of food consumed before eating fruits may impact your body's reaction. Foods that are high in protein, fiber, or fat would reduce the absorption rate of fruit nutrients into the body. Although, for those who are diabetics, this could be helpful because the sugars found in fruit would be slowly absorbed into the blood stream. This would be especially true for the most sugary or high glycemic fruits (to be discussed below).

Susan Mills-Gray, nutrition/health specialist at the University of Missouri Extension Center, has debunked this rotting theory. She rightfully points out that food does not rot in the stomach. She states that "while it is true that fruit is more quickly digested if it's the only food present in the stomach, the same is true for all food."

However, the fact still remains that the order of eating fruits may make a difference in the nutrient absorption rate. Mixing fruits with meals in your stomach does open an avenue for an array of chemical reactions. It has also been debated whether eating fruit first would actually cause gas and bloating.

This was addressed by Dr. Mark Pochapin, Professor of Gastroenterology and Professor of Medicine at the NYU School of Medicine, and Director of the Division of Gastroenterology at NYU Langone Medical Center. He says, "Rotting, or fermentation, means bacterial action on food resulting in decomposition. And because of the presence of hydrochloric acid, the stomach has very few bacteria. The place where fruit produces gas is in the colon, not the stomach."

Benefits of Eating Fruits Before Meals

Aside from all the speculation, there are true/ proven benefits to eating fruits before main meals.

Feeling full/ no binge eating

Fruits contain fiber. The digestive system does not break down fiber in the same way that it breaks down other foods during the digestion process. Fiber has bulk. This bulk creates a feeling of fullness and can help in controlling weight and not overeating.

When fruit is consumed on an empty stomach, there

is time for fiber to create a feeling of being full. However, when fruit is consumed after a meal or along with other foods, this additional benefit does not have time to transpire. Therefore, eating fruits some time prior to a meal may actually provide a long lasting feeling of fullness that results in not feeling hungry when it time for the next meal.

Anti-oxidant benefits

Most fruits are rich in antioxidants like lycopene, lutein and beta-carotene. Eating fruits before meals ensures your body takes full advantage of these antioxidants to free itself from harmful free radicals. Since free radicals are associated with and considered a prevailing cause of cancer, eating fruit before meals to receive the full benefit may be considered a way to help in the fight against cancer.

Advantage to diabetics

Fruits such as pears and apples tend to slow down the release of glucose into your bloodstream. This ultimately stabilizes your blood sugar level.

Maximum vitamins and minerals

To optimize on the rich properties, vitamins, and minerals of fruits, eating fruits before meals may serve as a primary tool. Vitamins and minerals in fruits are better absorbed on an empty stomach.

Before Exercising

Some fruits are good for consumption in small amounts before or in between exercise or physical training sessions. Fruits that are high in sugars or that contain higher rates of carbs will provide additional fuel to be burned during exercise. For example, bananas are a popular source of fuel for many athletes. It is common to see bananas during or at the end of marathons as a source of energy or to boost the blood sugar levels of runners who are running or have just completed the 26.2 mile race.

However, using "fruit fuel" for exercise may also result in a "fruit crash" if not replenished after a long period of exercise. Additionally, if the goal of exercise is weight loss, then it is always important to remember that fruits do contain some carbohydrates. The fuel from carbohydrates not burned off or used as fuel will eventually be converted into fat. So, the fruit or fuel consumed before exercise should be considered in combination with the exercise to be performed.

Fruits and Sugars

Many fruits contain natural sugars as a part of their composition. Now that more dieters understand the necessity of avoiding excess sugars, there seemingly is a growing push to avoid all fruits. The belief is that this will improve health and cause weight loss. However, it is important to fully consider this way of thinking. Just as 500 calories of vegetables are different than 500 calories of cookies or cake, there is a difference between the sugar in fruit and the sugars added to many of our foods today.

Has anyone become obese because of eating too many apples, blueberries, or strawberries?

Is eating 2 apples the same as drinking two 12 ounce sodas?

Are a handful of grapes the same as 8 ounces of grape soda?

Fruits contain natural sugars and also contain fiber. Although fiber will be covered in an upcoming chapter, it is important to point out a basic fact about fiber. Fiber is digested slowly and requires time for it to broken down. This is also true for the fiber in fruit.

The natural fructose in fruit *does* classify as a sugar. However, this sugar is not immediately processed the same as other simple sugars. It is released into the blood much more slowly. As such, consuming most fruits will not impact blood sugar the same way as it does with sugars from processed foods. Thus, most fruits will allow the blood sugar to rise much more slowly while also reaping the satisfying feeling of being full that comes with fiber.

So instead of avoiding all fruits like the plague, find comfort in going for that natural source of Vitamin C. If you are seeking that source from a juice version, however, you will need to be mindful of the amounts of sugar contained in the fruit you are drinking. Some fruit juices actually contain more sugar than sodas.

Glycemic Index for Fruits

There are loads of benefits that certain fruits may provide. Nevertheless, not all fruits are created equal. There are some fruits that it may be best to limit when considering weight loss and overall physical fitness. One way to know which fruits have less sugar than others is by utilizing the Glycemic Index.

You will want to avoid fruits with a High GI when trying to lose weight and not to over-indulge when not on a diet. The best fruits for weight loss and overall health are ones with a low Glycemic Index.

Average Glycemic Index (GI) scores

0-55 = Low GI

Cherries -	22	Prunes -	29
Plums -	24	Peach, canned - in natural juice	30
Grapefruit -	25		
Peaches -	28	Banana, - under ripe	30

Dried -	32	Pears	-	41
Apricots		Grapes	-	43
Apples -	34	Coconut -		45
Oranges -	40	Kiwi Fruit -		47
Strawberries -	40	Banana overripe -		52
Coconut Milk -	41			

56-69 = Medium GI

Sultanas -	56	Figs-	61
Apricot, raw -	57	Raisins -	64
Bananas -	58	Cantaloupes -	65
Mango -	60	Pineapple -	66
Papaya -	60	Pineapple -	66

70 or more = High GI

Watermelons -	80	Dates –	103

Fruits and weight loss

In addition to considering the GI, there may be a desire to lose weight by cutting out carbohydrates or limiting carbohydrates to a particular amount for each day. Carbohydrates do play an important part in the body's function. So, cutting out all carbs permanently may be another aspect of dieting in which it may be best to consult a doctor before going to any extremes.

There are those who are on a mission to lose weight by reducing their carbohydrate intake temporarily or permanently. If this is a goal, there are actually a number of high-carb fruits that may need to be removed from consideration. It may be important to find a fruit that will not spike blood sugar and that will not introduce excess glucose into the bloodstream.

Examples of high carbohydrate fruits include:

Peeled avocado (18g)
Apples (21g)
Dried apricots (24.9g)
Sweet bananas (23.7g)
Dried currants (26.7g)
Seedless Raisins (32.6g)
Dried figs (32.7g)
Chopped dates (32.7g)
Avocado (340 g)

For those who want to minimize their daily caloric intake, here are a couple of examples of low carbohydrate fruits:

Cantaloupe (14 g)
Strawberries (11 g)
Raspberries (15 g)
Papaya (14 g)
Honeydew Melon (15 g)
Fresh Apricots (17 g)

Find the nutritional value of your favorite fruits.

	Calories	Carbs	Fiber	Protein
		(g)	(g)	(g)
Apple	130	34	5	1
1 large				
Avocado	50	3	1	1
California,				
1/5 medium				
Banana	110	30	3	1
1 medium				
Cantaloupe	50	12	1	1
1/4 medium				
Grapefruit	60	15	2	1
1/2 medium				
Grapes	90	23	1	0
3/4 cup				
Honeydew Melon	50	12	1	1
1/10 medium melon				

Kiwifruit 2 medium	90	20	4	1
Lemon 1 medium	15	5	2	0
Lime 1 medium	20	7	2	0
Nectarine 1 medium	60	15	2	1
Orange 1 medium	80	19	3	1
Peach 1 medium	60	15	2	1
Pear 1 medium	100	26	6	1
Pineapple 2 slices,	50	13	1	1
Plums 2 medium	70	19	2	1

Strawberry	50	11	2	1
8 medium				
Sweet Cherries	100	26	1	1
21 cherries; 1 cup				
Tangerine	50	13	2	1
1 medium				
Watermelo n	80	21	1	1
1/18 medium melon;				

6

Vegetables

It is often stated time and time again that it is important to eat your 5 daily servings of vegetables. Why do vegetables play such an important part in our overall health? The fact that they are entirely natural and not processed is a huge factor in this analysis. Vegetables are considered to be living food, in that they are rich in vitamins and nutrients. Some vegetables contain so few calories that it is possible to have a plate full with little caloric intake. As such, vegetables are an essential ingredient when considering foods that are good for weight loss.

Vegetables do not have to be bland and boring with little flavor. It is good to know how to prepare them right to get the best taste and health benefits. Teamed with something you already enjoy eating and vegetables can suddenly become delicious.

The regular consumption of vegetables in our day to day eating regimen coupled with scheduled and intentional exercises may be the secret to your overall fitness.

The Secret Power of Vegetables

It is well understood that our bodies need a daily supply of vitamins, minerals, and components for fuel that allow them to run well. In fact, the daily consumption of vegetables helps to facilitate the smooth functioning of the body in a variety of ways.

Whether by preventing negative reactions or by promoting positive responses in the body, vegetables may be the most important food group. The preventative abilities of vegetables can greatly benefit us our health. Vegetables help reduce blood pressure and cholesterol levels, which can help protect against heart disease. They contain high levels of fiber and roughage that work tremendously in the proper digestion of food within the intestines, helping to cleanse your body from the inside.

Some vegetables contain antioxidants that are associated with the treatment and reduction of the probability of certain cancers. The nutrients present in vegetables also support and play important roles with diabetes, skin care, bone conditions, cardiovascular health, and intestinal health. Some of this occurs because minerals in vegetables assist in shielding our cells from unnecessary oxidation due to the presence of potassium, zinc, magnesium and other minerals in the body.

Additionally, vegetables are vital in that they contain phytonutrients – a chemical that is responsible for protecting and helping our bodies with a number of crucial ailments and diseases, such as cancer, asthma, and the fight against inflammation. Some examples of these defense phytonutrients are carotenoids and flavonoids, which are represented by the color of the vegetables. For example, green vegetables are excellent sources of fighting iron-related deficiencies.

Carbohydrates and Proteins in Vegetables

Most foods contain some measurable amount of carbs. Vegetables serve as a source of both carbohydrates and proteins. Many vegetables, however, contain what are described as "complex carbs." Complex carbs (as previously mentioned in the discussion on carbohydrates) are better than the common carbs generally found in breads, pastas, and processed foods. Complex carbs have more vitamins and do not quickly raise blood sugar levels like "sugary" simple carbs. Complex carbohydrates also possess fiber and some protein, too.

While the carbohydrates in vegetables are better than simple sugary carbs, there are some that may be highly loaded in carbs. For example, white potatoes are considered by many as being overly loaded with carbs, not easily be burned off, and therefore, fattening.

Meanwhile, foods like dried beans (often referred to as 'the poor man's meat') have the capacity to furnish the body with vital nutrients, promote weight loss, and hold off hunger. Many vegetables contain significant amounts of carbohydrates that do not promote weight gain. Some of these include carrots, beetroots, and yams.

The Best Time To Eat Vegetables

With all the different types of vegetables, it may be confusing when trying to figure out when the best time to eat the vegetables is and what vegetables should be eaten. Due to the amazing qualities in vegetables, they can be eaten all day long. Nevertheless, they are usually eaten during lunches and dinners rather than breakfasts. That is not to say that they cannot be eaten in the morning, but you can get most of your nutrients in your breakfast from other foods such as fruits and oats.

Eating vegetables throughout the day helps to evenly supplement the vital vitamins that are needed in the body. This may also help with keeping your energy levels up during the day and maintaining a level blood sugar. That notwithstanding, there are those who religiously prefer eating a bigger portion of them either at breakfast or during lunch time.

Breakfast

The rationale for loading on veggies early in the day is that since breakfast is the most important meal of the day, you can get your day started on a good note. For some, this equates to eating a meal that has a good amount of carbohydrates and fibers, with a little bit of proteins. Others prefer to take smaller amounts of vegetables in the morning as they incorporate other items and snack on vegetables between main meals.

Lunch

A downside to front loading the day with vegetables in the morning is that it leaves you vulnerable to overeating other high calorie foods throughout the rest of the day. Not feeling hunger throughout the day is essential to ensuring that you do not binge on sugary snacks that you and your body do not need.

Vegetables help provide a sense of satiety or feeling full because they can be consumed in higher quantities without a higher caloric intake. So, spreading out calories during the day may mean reducing calories over the course of the entire day as well. This would require eating vegetables for lunch and then dinner. A lunch full of vegetables may last until dinner and prevent someone from eating too much for dinner.

Dinner

Evening dinner is something that must be a part of a long-term workable diet. For those who enjoy having a full-size dinner, but are not able to burn off all the calories burned, a plate full of vegetables may be a great option. Because vegetables are naturally low in calories, vegetables as the primary food at dinner allows for satisfaction without weight gain. The food may be burned off quickly but provide a feeling of being full throughout the evening.

Dieting, at times, may feel create the feeling of being anti-social because of not being able to fully join in on the fun of eating. Vegetables, however, may serve as an appetizer priced alternative. You may be able to participate without having to join in with the weighted protein or carb loaded starches.

There are even a variety of options with vegetables for dinner. If you include meat with your dinner, the general rule however is 1/3 meat (or whatever else you are eating) mixed with 2/3 vegetables to make up a mostly green plate. As long as you are sure to add in your vegetables, you can choose the vegetables you like and learn to love them. However, power veggies like broccoli are always good choices.

Snacks

There are some vegetables that have the unique characteristics of burning more calories during consumption than they contain themselves. These vegetables still produce the satiating effect whereby one feels full for longer. Vegetables like spinach, watercress, celery and cucumber provide this benefit. They can be eaten raw or used as toppings on sandwiches. These vegetables will work as great snacks.

In addition to raw carrots as a vegetable snack option that can be eaten throughout the day, green leaf smoothies are also a viable option. These smoothies can be made by mixing your favorite vegetables like spinach, romaine lettuce, kale, and/or celery together in a blender. It is also an option to add fruits like blueberries, pineapples, and lemons for added flavor and sweetening. The end result will be a liquid concoction of your liking that will have amazing health benefits and keep you full.

Salads

A great day to day healthy lunch option is a salad with a variety of vegetables. A few options to add to a plate full of greens may be beans, tomatoes (sundried or fresh), seeds, or fruit to suit your own taste buds. However, the eater should be aware of what is being consumed.

Beware, the most popular salad dressings can cause a major setback in weight loss. The ingredients used in many dressings contain high levels of sugars and calories. Dressings that include ingredients such as mayonnaise and other fat-ridden condiments can serve as a key to turning a healthy salad into a green, high-calorie dessert.

It is helpful to read the labels of salad dressings to see what your dressings contain. Otherwise, you could be undoing all the hard work from eating properly and exercising, all due to calories in the salad dressing alone. Vinegar or vinaigrettes are a great choice to give your food some flavor without being fattening. Another great option is to add olive oil as a way to soften the crunchy freshness of vegetables.

* *

Quick Tip

The website myfooddiary.com suggests for serving sizes:

1 cup green salad	=	a baseball or a fist
1 baked potato	=	a fist
3/4 cup tomato juice	=	a small styro-foam cup
1/2 cup cooked	=	a scoop of ice cream
broccoli	=	or a light bulb

* * * * * * * * * * * * * * * * * * * *

Livestrong.com suggests that when trying to determine portions:

1. Your **fist** determines your **veggie** portions.

2. Your **palm** determines your **protein** portions.

3. Your **cupped hand** determines your **carbohydrate** portions.

4. Your **thumb** determines your **fat** portions.

* *

Daily Vegetable Preparation

Serving Size

Often, a confusing aspect of eating vegetables is not only choosing what to eat, but also knowing how much to eat. The United Stated Department of Agriculture recommends eating 5 servings of vegetables each day (as previously noted). However, most people cannot accurately dip into a dish and measure a serving unless there is always a measuring cup accessible. Most people will have to estimate what appears to be a serving when preparing their meal. Some resources provide help in estimating serving size.

How To Prepare Vegetables

The way that vegetables are cooked/prepared makes a big difference in the way that they taste. In some cases, it will also impact the benefits the vegetables will maintain. Also, once vegetables are no longer fresh, their value diminishes.

The most beneficial way to eat vegetables is raw. This ensures that all their minerals and vitamins are maintained. This is not possible with all types of vegetables, but some may be eaten raw: such as tomatoes, carrots, cucumbers, beets, nuts, seeds. (Even broccoli if you don't mind it a little crunchy!) A thorough washing is also encouraged especially if they are to be consumed raw.

Cooking Vegetables

Most vegetables actually taste better cooked. It is absolutely important to note that vegetables are very delicate and can easily lose their nutritional worth when subjected to extreme levels of heat or left uneaten for long periods. For those that must be cooked, light steaming is advisable to make certain that the nutrients are not wasted away through prolonged periods of high temperatures.

The color, texture, taste and benefits of vegetables are better retained when steamed. If you do not have a steamer, purchasing one may be an investment in your health. Otherwise, preparing vegetables stovetop, without grease, and with less heat than frying, may serve as an option.

Boiling

When vegetables are totally immersed in water and boiled, the water may absorb many of the nutrients away from the vegetables and into the water. Then, the only way to receive the full nutrient content is to use the excess water to prepare soups, instead of pouring it out.

Microwaving

By far, the **ABSOLUTE** worst way to prepare vegetables is by microwaving them. In microwaving vegetables, many nutrients are extinguished and what is left is a nutrient poor substance that does not possess the value expected or desired when eating vegetables. Unless there is no other option and you are opposed to cold veggies, avoid the microwave.

Fresh versus Canned Vegetables

Just as the manner in which vegetables are prepared may impact the nutritional quality, so will the means by which the vegetables are stored. This may play a major role in deciding what vegetables to eat. It may not always be practical to eat vegetables that are fresh out of the garden. Often, food will be frozen or canned as a means of storage. The added salt may also be a negative, if not properly rinsed.

Canned foods are able to withstand room

temperature for extended periods of time. They also may be easier to cook. However, there are additives such as salt included in the canning process that may reduce the full health benefits of the vegetables in their unadulterated state.

Frozen foods are a much better option. While there may be some reduction in the full nutritional value, fewer additives are necessary to maintain the freshness of the vegetables. There may be some drying from the freezing process. However, in comparison to being canned, frozen vegetables are a definite winner.

As always, it is important to read the labels of the package to learn what, if anything, has been included in the packaging process.

Which Vegetables To Choose

Not all vegetables have the same shape and color. They all have different qualities and taste completely different. Like any food group, vegetables have a variety of tastes and textures. If you are one of those people who says "I don't like vegetables," perhaps you have not tried a wide variety. So, before canceling out eating any vegetables and looking for vitamins as an alternative, a trip down to your local farmers market may be a worthwhile trip.

Dark green vegetables provide a multitude of vitamins. They are even linked to living longer, along with orange vegetables like squash.

Dry peas and beans are natural weight loss vegetables. They have a unique taste that many people enjoy.

Starchy vegetables such as sweet potatoes and corn are higher in calories than others, but they also have a wide range of vitamins.

In a nutshell, vegetables are an essential component of a healthy diet. They are best eaten fresh and from rainbow of colors - green, yellow, orange, purple, etc. Have a look online and in recipe books for vegetable dishes and give them a try. You might be pleasantly surprised at the new tastes that you discover. The more colorful, the better variety of nutrients to be consumed as a part of your regular diet.

Commonly eaten vegetables

Dark Green Vegetables

bok choy
broccoli
collard greens
dark green leafy
lettuce
kale

mustard greens
romaine lettuce
spinach
turnip greens
watercress

Starchy vegetables

cassava
corn
fresh cowpeas
 field peas
black-eyed peas (not
dry)
green bananas

green peas
green lima beans
plantains
potatoes
taro
water chestnuts

Red & orange vegetables

acorn squash
butternut squash
carrots
hubbard squash
pumpkin

red peppers
sweet potatoes
tomatoes
tomato juice

Beans and peas

black beans
black-eyed peas
(mature, dry)
garbanzo beans
(chickpeas)
kidney beans

lentils
navy beans
pinto beans
soy beans
split peas
white beans

Other vegetables

artichokes
asparagus
avocado
bean sprouts
beets
Brussels sprouts
cabbage
cauliflower
celery
cucumbers

eggplant
green beans
green peppers
iceberg (head) lettuce
mushrooms
okra
onions
turnips
wax beans
zucchini

Nutritional Value of popular vegetables

Vegetables	Calories	Carbs	Fiber	Protein
Serving Size				
(gram weight/ ounce weight)		(g)	(g)	(g)
Asparagus	20	4	2	2
5 spears				
Bell Pepper	25	6	2	1
1 medium				
Broccoli	45	8	3	4
1 medium stalk				
Carrot	30	7	2	1
1 carrot, 7" long, 1 1/4" diameter				
Cauliflower	25	5	2	2
1/6 medium head				
Celery	15	4	2	0
2 stalks				

Cucumber	10	2	1	1
1/3 medium				
Green (Snap) Beans	20	5	3	1
3/4 cup cut				
Green Cabbage	25	5	2	1
1/12 medium head				
Green Onion	10	2	1	0
1/4 cup chopped				
Iceberg Lettuce	10	2	1	1
1/6 medium head				
Leaf Lettuce	15	2	1	1
1 1/2 cups shredded				
Mushrooms	20	3	1	3
5 medium				

Onion 1 medium	45	11	3	1
Potato 1 medium	110	26	2	3
Radishes 7 radishes	10	3	1	0
Summer Squash 1/2 medium	20	4	2	1
Sweet Corn kernels from 1 medium ear	90	18	2	4
Sweet Potato 1 medium, 5" long, 2" diameter	100	23	4	2
Tomato 1 medium	25	5	1	1

7

Muscle Building Protein

Proteins are part of 3 primary groups of nutrients (proteins, carbohydrates, vitamins/ minerals). Proteins are large molecules made up of several chains of amino acids which are essential to the functioning of the body.

What Are Proteins Good For?

Protein is the second most plentiful molecule in the human body, next to water. In understanding the important role that protein plays in the proper functioning of our bodies, it becomes obvious how important it is that a healthy diet includes protein. When protein is consumed and digested, it is converted into amino acids. These amino acids are then broken down to promote the body's proper operation and functioning.

Proteins have a wide range of functions that can be

carried out in a variety of ways.

1. Proteins provide support to cells, the building blocks of the body, by helping them to form their structure and to operate properly.

2. Proteins work as antibodies that defend the body against foreign entities.

3. Proteins serve as enzymes that are responsible for numerous chemical reactions in cells and aid in forming new molecules.

4. Proteins may operate as hormones which are messenger proteins which help regulate activities in the body.

5. Carrier proteins move other molecules around the body, i.e. hemoglobin.

6. Protein contributes to the contraction of muscles. Additionally, skin, bones, organs, blood, hormones, tendons, and muscles are all comprised of protein.

Sources of Protein

The sources of protein are typically divided into two categories:

A) Animal Sources

B) Plant Sources

Animal Sources

Animal sources have the highest concentration of protein per gram. They also are better sources of essential amino acids, as compared to plant sources. Animal sources include red meat, white meat (that includes chicken and fish), eggs, mutton, and milk and dairy products. Of the animal sources, meat is a major protein source for those in the Americas and Western culture due to its availability and a long tradition of consuming meat. However, choosing the wrong meat for protein can result in negative consequences.

Too much Red Meat

In the effort to consume proteins (or from a love of steak and burgers), many meat eaters find themselves eating a high amount of red meat. However, consumption of too much red meat may cause a large number of complications, such as an increased risk of cardiovascular disease. Some proteins contain large amounts of saturated fats that have been associated with cardiovascular and heart disease. This is especially the case with processed red meat.

Even though slight, small amounts of processed red meat can have a great impact on the risk of dying from cardiovascular disease. Just an additional 1.5

ounce serving each day has been associated with a 20 percent greater risk of cardiovascular death. That is the equivalent of one hot dog or two strips of bacon each day.

Also, some red meat is high in cholesterol and can easily lead to obesity, which may cause a host of other complications. It is not necessarily the meat that is poor for health but the additional saturated fats that are included. For example, a 6 ounce broiled porterhouse steak may contribute 60 percent of the recommended daily intake of saturated fat for someone eating a 2,000 calorie per day diet, all in one meal.

* *

Quick Tip

It is not only the saturated fat that may be detrimental to health. It may be sodium or cancer causing nitrates contained in the food.

* *

The main alternatives to red meat are chicken, fish, and beans. It has been found that substituting these alternatives in place of red meat reduces the risks of cardiovascular disease associated with red meat. In fact, chicken and fish have twice as less cholesterol as red meat. Additionally, fish meat is rich in Omega 3 oils which are good for the brain and for decreasing cholesterol.

Plant Sources

Plant substitutes and their products may also serve as an alternative to red meat. With these options, red meat can be completely eliminated from the diet which will be much healthier and will lower cholesterol. So, while animal meat may be a high source of protein, it may come with its consequences if one is not careful.

Most plant sources have lower concentrations of protein per gram. Thus, they have to be consumed in larger quantities than meat to attain the minimum Recommended Dietary Allowance of around 56 grams.

Plant sources include: peas, beans, soy beans and nuts like walnuts and almonds. Many vegetarians choose soybeans as a meat alternative. These beans can be grounded and turned into various products that would otherwise require an animal, such as milk and patties.

Whole grains and cereals also may serve as a source of protein when consumed. However, the value received is limited in comparison to other animal or plant based sources of protein. Additionally, vegetables that would be considered root vegetables are not good sources of protein.

Fruits also are considered a poor source of protein, despite their many other benefits. Nevertheless, a balanced diet or a diet that has been carefully thought out, will be filled with the appropriate amount of proteins.

Protein Supplements and Manufactured Protein Sources

In recent years, there has been a rapid increase in the number of protein supplements such as protein bars and shakes. These supplements serve to take the place of protein that might be consumed from animal and plant sources. They also come packaged in a variety of ways that make them easy to carry and consume without any preparation or cooking.

These supplements provide the opportunity for easy consumption. However, it must be remembered that what is consumed is a modified version of protein that is not naturally found in nature. Thus, it is often debated whether this processed protein is as rich and plentiful as animal and plant based protein sources.

One major unintended consequence of consuming protein products is that one must consume all the other ingredients that are contained in the bar or shake. For instance, no one desires to eat a protein bar that tastes bad. So, manufacturers include numerous additives to make their product an enjoyable experience. In order to achieve this goal, products often have sugars added, are high in calories, or contain other additives that any manufactured ingredients. Meanwhile, the actual amount of protein included may not always be as high as desired for the amount of calories being consumed.

Dr. (Emmett) Oz suggested that when shopping for protein bars, make sure that 4 requirements have been met.

1. It has at least 10 grams of protein.
2. It has less than 15 grams of sugar (the lower, the better).
3. It has less than 4 grams of fat – and no trans-fats allowed.
4. It has less than 350 calories.

Finding bars that meet these four requirements may not always be easily accomplished. This is especially true when the goal is to lose weight.

Protein assists many bodily functions like building muscle. Most bodybuilders take advantage of the convenience protein shakes and bars in their effort to build muscle. If you are already consuming a significant amount of protein from a regularly balanced diet, eating a protein bar that contains extra calories may not be necessary if the desire is to lose weight.

Finding a pure source of protein that does not include all of the other ingredients may be a better option. If all else fails, a fruit like an apple may serve as an easy to carry alternative that does not require much preparation other than washing.

Protein for weight loss versus protein for muscle building

Protein can be used to either help a person lose weight, build muscle, or both at the same time. Muscles burn more calories than fat. So, developing lean muscle mass that is not bulky can be an effective weight loss strategy. Also, a high protein diet, along with limiting the intake of carbs and sugars, can help a dieter to lose weight and suppress the appetite.

Proteins will help provide the feeling of being full, leading to a lower calorie intake throughout the day.

Calories of protein are superior (not as fat inducing) than calories of carbohydrates and sugars. Therefore, it is understandable that increasing proteins while limiting carbohydrates and sugars will help with losing weight. It is usually recommended that those wishing to lose weight using a high protein diet consume white meat, nuts and whole grains as their sources of protein due to their low saturated fat concentration.

A Harvard University study of 120,000 male and female subjects over a period of 20 years revealed that those who ate an increased number of nuts during the study gained less weight than those who consumed more red and processed meat. (It is important to drink plenty of water with nuts to assist the nuts with digestion and preventing them from feeling solid and like cement in one's stomach.)

For those wishing to build muscle, proteins are usually consumed shortly after working out because the muscle cells need to be repaired from the physical activity of weight lifting. A high protein diet promotes a fast recovery of muscle cells and their quick growth. It also reduces the need to consume protein supplements, and in some cases, eliminates the need to use them completely.

Best Times To Eat Protein

So, when is the best time to consume protein to lose weight and build muscle? For many foods the answer is, "it depends." *Apparently, for proteins the answer for when to eat them is, "whenever you can."*

When considering how much to consume each day, The Institute of Medicine recommends having 8 grams of protein for every 20 pounds of personal body weight. That would be about 80 grams of protein for a 200 pound man or 56 grams for a 140 pound female. There is also the suggestion that 10-35% of calories consumed be from protein. However, that can come from a variety of sources. When reading labels, one will easily discover that a calorie of protein is far more nutritious than a random calorie from carbohydrates or processed foods.

Additionally, high-protein, low-carbohydrate diets have been increasingly associated with weight loss and with improved health numbers. A 20 year study that included over 80,000 women found that such a high-protein, low-carbohydrate diet reduced the risk of heart disease by 30 percent. Another study found results that suggested a lower blood pressure and lower bad cholesterol (LDL). These results are ultimately because of the choice of protein sources that did not include other negatives.

So, what do we know are the keys to using proteins for improved health and weight management?

1. Having 5-6 meals, every 2-3 hours throughout the day help boost metabolism and prevents hunger.

2. Protein serves as a hunger suppressant.

3. Protein serves as a muscle builder, and muscles burn calories faster than fat.

4. Protein calories do not cause excess fat gain like calories from carbohydrates and sugars.

5. Protein may be good before and after exercise.

Breakfast

During our hours of sleep, the body uses nutrients already in the body for its regular functioning. So, what is consumed as a part of the first meal is critical in replenishing the body and setting the tone for the day going forward.

Breakfast meals have traditionally included foods that contain carbs and protein. Instead of looking for the carb loaded pancakes and sugary syrup, consider foods that are high in protein.

Now there are a variety of options that may depend

on your preferences or dietary restrictions such as:

Fruit,

milk (animal or plant based),

eggs (boiled or scrambled),

yogurt (non-sugary),

sausage/ bacon (turkey or pork), or

a muscle building shake.

Lunch

For protein, lunch may include a mix of foods that are easily digested. This protein will be slowly released or stay in the stomach for some time. White meat such as chicken and fish are ideal for lunch, as they are not as heavy as red meat. At the same time, they remain in the stomach for some time, preventing a feeling of hunger. However, if the goal is to stay away from meats, alternatives such as legumes, beans, and nuts are also sources of protein for lunch or for a snack. They are low in calories and provide a feeling of satiety as well.

Dinner

The dinner options may be similar to those for lunch. However, there will not be as much time to burn off the calories before bedtime. So, this may be the time to consider foods that are low calorie and provide a feeling of being full. Use protein to help fight late the night snacking temptations that often bring us down.

Commonly eaten protein foods

Meats*

Lean cuts of:

beef	pork
ham	veal
lamb	

Game Meats

bison	venison
rabbit	

Lean Ground Meats

beef	lamb
pork	

Organ Meats

liver	giblets

Poultry

chicken
duck
goose
turkey

ground chicken and
turkey
eggs
chicken eggs
duck eggs

Beans and Peas

bean burgers
black beans
black-eyed peas
chickpeas (garbanzo
beans)
falafel
kidney beans

lentils
lima beans (mature)
navy beans
pinto beans
soy beans
split peas
white beans

Processed Soy Products

tofu (bean curd made
from soybeans)
veggie burgers

tempeh
texturized vegetable
protein (TVP)

Nuts and Seeds

almonds
cashews
hazelnuts (filberts)
mixed nuts
peanuts
peanut butter

pecans
pistachios
pumpkin seeds
sesame seeds
sunflower seeds
walnut

Seafood

Finfish such as:

catfish
cod
flounder
haddock
halibut
herring
mackerel
pollock

porgy
salmon
sea bass
snapper
swordfish
trout
tuna

Shellfish such as:

clams
crab
crayfish
lobster
mussels

octopus
oysters
scallops
squid (calamari)
shrimp

Canned fish such as:

anchovies
clams

tuna
sardines

8

Fiber

Fiber is a nutrient that is found in many fruits, vegetables, beans and whole grains. Foods that are rich in fiber often have the benefit of being low in calories but rank high in preventing hunger.

As a complex carbohydrate, fiber is not easily digestible. As it works its way through the intestines and digestive tract, it is able to collect other items that have not been digested. Fiber forces these materials through the digestive system for disposal. Through this process, fiber can serve as a useful tool in the weight loss process. In addition to weight loss, fiber serves to prevent many digestive illnesses, hemorrhoids, and even colon cancer.

There are many foods contain fiber. They can be separated into two different categories: soluble and insoluble. Fruits, vegetables, and beans that are high in fiber assist the body to decrease bad cholesterol levels and also help in balancing blood-sugar levels. These dissolvable types of fiber are categorized as soluble. Other sources of fiber, like whole grains, serve as a natural laxative and help to cleanse the body as a natural digestive detoxification source. These non-dissolvable sources of fiber are categorized as being insoluble.

Soluble fiber dissolves in water and assists the body in a variety of ways. Soluble fiber may help regulate the digestive system. It has been found to promote a decrease in bad cholesterol (LDL) levels, stabilize blood sugar, lower the risk of heart disease, and reduce the risk of type 2 diabetes. It can be found in a number of plant based foods.

Examples of soluble fiber include:

apples	peas
apricots	oatmeal
beans	oat bran
blueberries	oranges
brussels	nuts
flaxseeds	pears
grapefruit	sprouts
lentils	strawberries
mangoes	whole grain
oranges	

Insoluble fiber does not dissolve in water and will maintain some size because it is not broken down as much as soluble fiber. As such, insoluble fiber primarily benefits digestive system by serving as a natural laxative and helping to cleanse the body as a natural digestive detoxification source. It assists in cleansing out materials from the digestive tract that were not previously excreted. As a result, this type of fiber also works to prevent diverticulitis disease (the build-up of tiny pockets along the lining of the colon).

Examples of insoluble fiber include:

barley	nuts
brown rice	raisins
carrots	seeds
celery	tomatoes
cucumbers	wheat bran
dark leafy vegetables	whole grains
grapes	zucchini
green beans	

When To Eat Fiber

Getting the right amount of fiber in your diet may take planning and intentional effort. The average adult only consumes about 15 grams. For women, the recommended daily intake amount of fiber is 25 grams a day; for men, 35-40.

So, should fiber be eaten at particular points during the day to get the most out of it? *Fiber can be eaten whenever you want. A little bit with every meal is helpful, if you can manage it.* However, if you are striving for weight loss or fitness, then eating your fiber during specifically planned times can be a useful tool.

Fiber in the morning is great to give you an energy boost for the day ahead and to maintain blood sugar levels. All bran or oats are great options for breakfast, perhaps topped with raspberries, which also have a high amount of fiber. Many foods that are packed with fiber are filling and will help fight off hunger. So, in addition to including fiber with breakfast, it may prove beneficial to having a fiber-rich snack.

Because of the digestive aid that fiber provides, it may be tempting to time fiber intake with a preferred time for using the bathroom. However, everyone's digestive system is different, and it may not be as predictable as a scheduling a flight. It may be difficult to predict a regular timeline for passing whatever various foods that have been accumulated in one's digestive tract.

Instead of trying to find the perfect time for fiber, it is more important to take the time to find ways for fiber to be a regular part of your diet. Many foods that are rich in proteins are also good fiber sources. Therefore, there may be an opportunity to use one food for two purposes.

With Exercise?

It is also a good idea to consider when to eat fiber when planning for exercising. Because of the role fiber plays in passing food, choosing when to consume fiber can be vital to an effective exercise session or having to run to the bathroom. Many runners have experienced GI (gastro-intestinal) distress during a run after having consumed foods high in fiber. Consuming fiber near the time of their run has caused many runners to experience diarrhea (also known as runner's trots or giving runners the runs). If working out in the morning, it may be best to hold off on the fiber until after the workout.

Meanwhile, if the plan is to exercise in the afternoon, whether your lunch was filled with fiber is something to consider. A fiber-rich snack a few hours before an afternoon workout may be manageable, and it will provide the benefit of preventing hunger during the workout. If you notice much GI distress during or after your exercise sessions, it may be helpful to evaluate the timing of your fiber consumption.

Find the amounts of fiber in various foods in the list below and in the Appendix.

Foods High In Both Protein and Fiber

Description	Protein (g) Per 100 g	Fiber, total dietary (g) Per 100 g	Carbs, by difference (g) Per 100 g
Beans, black turtle, mature seeds, raw	21.25	15.5	63.25
Beans, black, mature seeds, raw	21.6	15.5	62.36
Beans, cranberry (roman), mature seeds, raw	23.03	24.7	60.05
Beans, XXXrench, mature seeds, raw	18.81	25.2	64.11
Beans, great northern, mature seeds, raw	21.86	20.2	62.37

Beans, kidney, all types, mature seeds, raw	23.58	24.9	60.01
Beans, navy, mature seeds, raw	22.33	24.4	60.75
Beans, pink, mature seeds, raw	20.96	12.7	64.19
Beans, pinto, mature seeds, raw	21.42	15.5	62.55
Beans, small white, mature seeds, raw	21.11	24.9	62.25
Beans, white, mature seeds, raw	23.36	15.2	60.27
Beans, yellow, mature seeds, raw	22	25.1	60.7
Broadbeans , mature seeds, raw	26.12	25	58.29

Chickpeas (garbanzo beans, bengal gram), mature seeds, raw	19.3	17.4	60.65
Chives, freeze-dried	21.2	26.2	64.29
Corn, dried, yellow (Northern Plains Indians)	14.48	20.5	66.27
Cowpeas, common (blackeyes, crowder, southern), mature seeds, raw	23.52	10.6	60.03
Hazelnuts, beaked (Northern Plains Indians)	14.89	9.8	22.98
Hyacinth beans, mature seeds, raw	23.9	25.6	60.74

Lentils, raw	25.8	30.5	60.08
Lima beans, large, mature seeds, raw	21.46	19	63.38
Lima beans, thin seeded (baby), mature seeds, raw	20.62	20.6	62.83
Lupins, mature seeds, raw	36.17	18.9	40.37
Nuts, almond butter, plain, without salt added	20.96	10.3	18.82
Nuts, almonds	21.15	12.5	21.55
Nuts, almonds, dry roasted, w/o salt added	20.96	10.9	21.01
Nuts, almonds, honey roasted, unblanched	18.17	13.7	27.9

Nuts, almonds, oil roasted, without salt added	21.23	10.5	17.68
Nuts, hazelnuts or filberts	14.95	9.7	16.7
Nuts, hazelnuts or filberts, dry roasted, without salt added	15.03	9.4	17.6
Nuts, pine nuts, pinyon, dried	11.57	10.7	19.3
Nuts, pistachio nuts, dry roasted, without salt added	20.95	9.9	29.38
Nuts, pistachio nuts, raw	20.27	10.3	27.51
Oat bran, raw	17.3	15.4	66.22

Oats	16.89	10.6	66.27
Parsley, freeze-dried	31.3	32.7	42.38
Peanuts, all types, oil-roasted, without salt	28.03	9.4	15.26
Peanuts, spanish, raw	26.15	9.5	15.82
Peas, split, mature seeds, raw	24.55	25.5	60.37
Peppers, ancho, dried	11.86	21.6	51.42
Peppers, hot chile, sun-dried	10.58	28.7	69.86
Peppers, pasilla, dried	12.35	26.8	51.13
Pigeon peas (red gram), mature seeds, raw	21.7	15	62.78
Seeds, chia seeds, dried	16.54	34.4	42.12

Seeds, flaxseed	18.29	27.3	28.88
Seeds, pumpkin and squash seeds, whole, roasted, without salt	18.55	18.4	53.75
Seeds, sesame butter, tahini, from raw and stone ground kernels	17.81	9.3	26.19
Seeds, sesame butter, tahini, from roasted and toasted kernels (most common type)	17	9.3	21.19
Seeds, sesame seed kernels, dried (decorticated)	20.45	11.6	11.73
Seeds, sesame seed kernels, toasted, w/out salt (decorticated)	16.96	16.9	26.04

Seeds, sesame seeds, whole, dried	17.73	11.8	23.45
Seeds, sesame seeds, whole, roasted and toasted	16.96	14	25.74
Seeds, sunflower seed kernels, dry roasted, without salt	19.33	11.1	24.07
Seeds, sunflower seed kernels, oil roasted, without salt	20.06	10.6	22.89
Seeds, sunflower seed kernels, toasted, without salt	17.21	11.5	20.59
Soybeans, mature seeds, raw	36.49	9.3	30.16
Soybeans, mature seeds, roasted, no			

salt added	35.22	17.7	33.55
Tomatoes, sun-dried	14.11	12.3	55.76
Winged beans, mature seeds, raw	29.65	25.9	41.71
Yardlong beans, mature seeds, raw	24.33	11	61.91

9

Not When, But
How Much Water

Many people commonly know that our bodies are made up of approximately 70% water. Parts of your body that you may not even consider contain water. Things like bones, fingernails, and hair all have a percentage of water content. While this makes the need for and benefits of water drinking somewhat obvious, we often find ourselves failing to stay properly hydrated.

How much water?

A lack of water in your diet will present some common issues such as dry skin and hair, headaches, and other health related issues. It is often suggested that the golden rule to drinking water is to have at least 8 cups of 8 ounces of water daily. That information seems to have originated with a 1945 recommendation by the Food and Nutrition Board. Based on its calculations of a daily calorie intake of 1900 calories, it utilized a formula that suggested 64 ounces of water each day. Since then, it has been adopted by most people as the solid truth. However, it is now somewhat inaccurate according to new and more detailed research.

The Institute of Medicine has now established new recommended guidelines for water intake. Science has shown that body type, sex, and age all play a role in how much water you actually need. Physical activity will also have a significant role in the appropriate amount of daily water consumption. Active people will require more water than those who are relatively inactive to replenish what is sweated out of the body. Those who are inactive should still work to reach the suggested daily minimum as well. (Of course, they should also work to become more active!)

Likewise, there are a number of other factors that may affect someone's recommended water intake. For example, the environment where you live may impact how much water is most appropriate for you. Hot or humid weather may impact someone's intake of fluid. As with exercise, these weather conditions can result in someone naturally sweating to stay cool, even if not active. Health conditions may also necessitate additional water for proper hydration. Pregnancy, breast feeding, and illnesses that cause diarrhea or vomiting will also require an increased intake of water because of how the fluid within the body is being redirected or released.

When there are no unique conditions, the Institute of Medicine finds that an average female requires approximately 91 ounces of water each day and approximately 125 ounces of water daily for men. This amount includes all sources of fluid. Nearly 80 percent of this intake can come from water and other drinks. Twenty percent of the daily fluid intake may come from foods.

Water for weight loss

While the daily fluid amount recommended by the Institute of Medicine includes all liquids, there is no comparison to the pure, unadulterated benefits of water. One hundred ounces of pure water is much more beneficial than 100 ounces of sugar loaded soda. Even diet sodas have been found to have detrimental effects on the body. In fact, drinking water at the beginning of each meal is a proven strategy for weight loss.

A 12 week study by the American Chemical Society in Boston revealed that those who consumed two eight ounce glasses of water before a meals lost an average of 5 pounds more than those who did not. Maintaining such a regiment would result in a loss of 20 pounds over the course of a year period without even stepping onto a treadmill, elliptical, or doing any exercise.

Consuming water shortly after awakening may also be beneficial for overall health. This is because the time during which we sleep is essentially our longest period without food or liquid. Therefore, it is important to replenish our bodies when we awaken. This is one reason why breakfast is so essential in the morning. However, when taking into consideration the body's need to stay hydrated, it is even more important to re-hydrate early into the new day.

Cold water for weight loss

Drinking cold water is ideal as it provides a refreshing relief. However, it appears that using a cold water diet for weight loss will not provide many results on the scale quickly. Some diet plans have offered that drinking cold water (33-43 degrees Fahrenheit) actually burns calories in a way that will provide weight loss if done on a regular basis.

The premise is that cold water will reduce body's temperature and require energy to be used to return the body back to its original, core temperature. This fat is true. However, studies like those performed by Beth Kitchin, Ph.D. of the University of Alabama at Birmingham's School of Public Health, have indicated that the results are minimal. These minimal results reveal that approximately 4 calories may be burned per 18 ounces (518 mL). That would require almost 500 ice cold glasses of water to burn one (1) pound. Cold water may, however, serve as an aid to cool off the body after a heated workout.

There was a hoax being circulated that drinking cold water after a meal causes stomach cancer. This myth started when a false email spread throughout the internet. The theory proposed that cold water would cause toxic sludge to build up in the stomach. This information has been debunked. However, that will not prevent the rumor from being repeated.

Best time to drink water

There is little doubt that water is the best fluid you can drink throughout the day. Hydrating the body without any added calories or sugars is surpassed by nothing else. Water will assist you with weight loss, and help you maintain a healthy weight. In fact, lifestyle of regularly drinking water throughout the day may be considered a useful ingredient for a lifetime of great health.

10

Coffee

The diet and weight loss world wouldn't be the same without caffeine. Just about every diet pill contains caffeine. Pre-workout energy snacks are full of caffeine. Of course, nearly one billion people drink coffee worldwide for its stimulation. Next to water, coffee and tea are the most consumed beverages in the world. People enjoy both drinks around the world for the caffeine content, taste, and their numerous health benefits.

Benefits of Coffee

Each 8 fluid ounces serving of coffee contains 90-105 mg of caffeine. For most, the effects help you feel more alert and focused, while providing a boost of energy. Coffee in moderation includes health benefits, such as helping to reduce the likelihood of attaining certain diseases such as Parkinson's disease and certain types of cancer. Caffeine can stimulate metabolism and be used as a powerful weight loss enhancer. Moreover, drinking coffee before an exercise session may even serve as a source of energy and help to maintain focus when trying to have a productive workout.

When to Drink Coffee

Countless people around the world seek coffee as a morning jolt and motivation to get them going for the day ahead. Knowing that coffee will provide a caffeinated boost, there is often the desire to have it at the right time for the most ideal results. For some, they feel that it will take hours to get going without their daily dose of coffee. However, a poorly timed regular dose of morning coffee may actually cause a decrease in the effectiveness of the coffee's impact. So, instead of always reaching for that morning Cup of Joe for continuous focus throughout the day, it may be beneficial to find the best and most effective time of day for caffeinated success.

Peak hours

When you wake up in the morning, the body produces its own natural energy source to provide alertness - cortisol. This chemical is connected to and supports the body's natural circadian cycle and rhythm. It helps us get tired to go to sleep and then to awaken and become alert during the day.

Two studies suggest that there may be a peak in the release of cortisol between the (averaged) hours of 8:00 – 9:00 AM. This is similar to a natural shot of caffeine that originates from within the body itself. So, while caffeine at an earlier point of the day will aid in providing greater alertness, the effects may be dulled because of the natural addition of cortisol. In other words, most people will become more alert anyway, even without their regular dose of caffeine.

Not only is the stimulation that comes from drinking coffee shortly after waking up not the best time to get the most long lasting effect, but a tolerance may be built up over time as well. So, where one cup of coffee in the morning once provided a strong jolt, multiple cups of coffee become necessary to get the same benefit. This tolerance may then translate into a desire to refuel on caffeine throughout the day to get the same effect as in the past. As a result, the additional cups consumed for alertness may also come with the added sugars, creamers, and calories often used to flavor that coffee.

You may be different

The effect of cortisol may depend on exactly how early you are reaching for that morning coffee. It may also depend on the time of the year and the weather. The timing of cortisol being at peak release between 8:00 and 9:00 AM is not necessarily because of an internal clock. In fact, it is based on an outward clock – sunlight.

The introduction of sunlight has been found to be an environmental trigger that serves notice for cortisol to be released. Thus, it only makes sense that this timing may be adjusted for the time of year. In the late spring and summer when the sun rises earlier in the day, the release of cortisol may be earlier. Meanwhile, the dark mornings of winter may have a late sun rise and a corresponding later spike in cortisol. As such, if you are waking up and reaching for that cup of coffee on a cloud and dreary day, it has been debated whether that coffee would be better earlier.

Weight loss

For some, a morning coffee is actually a weight loss barrier. This is especially true when taking into consideration the various and creative ways that we are now able to consume our caffeine. Thanks to coffee shops like Starbucks, our morning caffeinating has become an expression of personal creativity. Whether iced or hot, with caramel or whip cream, mocha or espresso, we have found new ways to flavor that additional morning boost. These expressions of coffee creativity may actually serve as sources of extra calories that may contradict and inhibit the progress being made to lose weight.

Studies have suggested that a cup of coffee in the morning may actually create a craving for sweets. This is related to caffeine's effect on cortisol levels. Then, add into the discussion that most people prefer to add sugar to their coffee. It gets even worse when coffee is included with a sugary, simple carbohydrate treat like doughnuts or a white bread bagel.

* *

Quick Tip

Instead of believing that it is necessary to completely give up coffee, it may be enough to be aware of any cravings that follow. That way, instead of reaching for that favorite sugary treat, you can choose to reach for another appetite suppressing snack.

* *

A quick peek at a Starbucks menu serves as an example of how a desire to become caffeinated can equate to a calorie loading experience.

	Calories	Fat (g)	Carb. (g)	Fiber (g)	Protein
Caffè Latte	190	7	18	0	12
Caffè Mocha	260	8	42	2	13
Cappuccino	120	4	12	0	8
Caramel Flan Latte	250	6	37	0	11
Caramel Macchiato	240	7	34	0	10
Cinnamon Dolce Latte	260	6	40	0	11
Iced Hazelnut Macchiato	230	5	34	0	10
Iced Skinny Flavored Latte	110	4	12	0	7

Iced Vanilla Latte	190	4	30	0	7
Iced Vanilla Macchiato	230	6	35	0	10
Iced Vanilla Spice Latte	190	4	31	0	7
Iced White Chocolate Mocha	340	9	55	0	11
Pumpkin Spice Latte	310	6	49	0	14
Salted Caramel Mocha	330	8	61	2	12
Skinny Cinnamon Dolce Latte	180	6	18	0	12
Skinny Flavored Latte	180	6	18	0	12
Vanilla Latte	250	6	37	0	12
Vanilla Macchiato	230	6	33	0	10
Cinnamon Dolce Frappuccino® Blended Beverage	350	4.5	64	0	15
Double Chocolaty Chip Frappuccino® Blended Crème	500	9	98	3	14

Best (most effective) time of day for coffee

How someone prepares their coffee has become a form of personal expression. For some, it is proof of their American first Amendment right of freedom of expression. As such it is your right to choose how and when to drink coffee. So, the timing of drinking coffee will not be described as a best time of day option. Rather it will be considered from a point of effectiveness.

The most effective times of day to drink coffee for continued alertness may require that there be some delay from that initial cup of coffee. The hours of 9:30 -11:30 a.m. provide for increased and lasting stimulation when considered with releases of cortisol. Another round of caffeine after lunch, between 1:30 and 3:30 p.m., may also provide for effective results that last throughout the day. Beware of caffeine too late in the day, though. Drinking coffee after 5pm, however, can cause restlessness or trouble falling asleep.

Because everyone has different chemical make-ups and sleep schedules, this schedule will vary from person to person. The times given are a general guideline for a typical adult with a regular, daily sleep pattern.

11

Green Tea and other teas . . .

Green tea is also one of the healthiest drinks in the world due to all of its benefits. Green tea is an excellent source of caffeine. It will even help you lose weight if consumed often enough.

Weight and Health Benefits of Green Tea

By weight, green tea is 20-45% polyphenols and 60-70% of those polyphenols are free radical killing catechins. Free radicals are molecules, ions, and atoms that damage the healthy molecules in our bodies. The side effects of damage from free radicals are obesity, cancer, and numerous illnesses. Thus, the anti-oxidants found in green tea work to prevent these complications.

Polyphenols in green tea give it anti-inflammatory and anti-oxidant properties. Another benefit of polyphenols is the ability they give the liver and muscle cells to use more fatty acids for fuel. This action gives the body more energy and endurance for exercise. Also, the same polyphenols that help fight illness, reduce excess triglycerides that store in our body and turn into fat.

Epigallocatechin gallate (EGCG) is the most abundant catechin in green tea with health benefits that includes treatment for fatigue, HIV, cancer, and fatty acid synthase. The EGCG in green tea also stimulates metabolism and allows fat to enter the bloodstream. The body then burns the fat as fuel instead of storing it as body fat which lowers blood pressure, blood sugar levels, and improves the blood flow to the heart, lowering cholesterol.

EGCG has become one of the most popular dietary supplements in the last decade due to the metabolism stimulation and fat burning ability.

When to Drink Green Tea

Green tea contains about half as much caffeine as coffee at 25-45mg per serving. The lower caffeine content will allow you to consume more green tea than coffee and stay in a healthy range of caffeine intake. This allows you to drink 4-6 cups of green tea per day and receive all its other benefits.

The caffeine effects of green tea follow the same cortisol-release pattern of coffee. Best consumption times are 9:30 -11:00 a.m. and 1:30 -3:30 p.m., similar to coffee. However, with a lesser caffeine content, green tea could be consumed later in the day than coffee. Drinking too late but will still also have the same problems of consuming caffeine late in the day.

To retain the health benefits of green tea, avoid boiling at temperature of 160-180 degrees is recommended.

Other Tea Types and Benefits

Seasonal teas and other teas do not have quite the same health benefits as green tea. However, they may possess other positive qualities not associated with green tea. For example, the caffeine content is higher with black tea and some seasonal teas. These fermented teas allow the leaves to oxidize and lose some of the beneficial polyphenols. Unfermented white tea has the similar health benefits as green tea and with less caffeine. White tea contains 15-25 mg of caffeine per serving, and black tea contains 35-50 mg caffeine per serving.

Coffee and Tea Weight Loss Benefits

Coffee and green tea are both excellent to aid you in weight loss and exercise. The benefits of the caffeine will give you more focus, drive, and energy allowing you to work harder during exercise. Green tea has the benefit of polyphenols allowing essential acids to store in muscle cells and the liver which would make it a prime candidate for pre-exercise fuel. Coffee has more caffeine giving you more stimulation than the green tea.

Coffee and tea are healthier choices over energy drinks or caffeinated soda drinks. These other drinks provide caffeine, but they also contain high amounts of processed sugar. You will find no serious diet plan that suggests consuming soda. Diet versions exist, but they also contain artificial sweeteners linked to numerous health risks. So, if the stimulation of caffeine is desired, there is no doubt that it is better to seek out coffee and tea instead of other processed drinks.

12

Alcohol and Liquid Calories

Those who are highly focused on dieting and exercise are not considered as candidates for carelessly and regularly getting inebriated. Alcohol and weight loss generally are not subjects that go together. This may be because of the conflicting lifestyle that they present. Those who are maintaining a regular exercise routine will often find that too much alcohol may reduce someone's motivation and energy levels necessary for the next day's work out. Also, alcoholic beverages are often considered to be liquid calories that do not serve a specific dietary or nutritional purpose. Thus, alcohol almost equates to excess weight.

There are some known benefits that are commonly associated with drinking in moderation. For instance, in red wine, there are benefits such as improved blood flow, insulin sensitivity, cardiovascular health, and anti-aging properties. Also, when it comes to consuming an alcoholic beverage or other sugary drinks like sodas and other sweetened fruit juices, there is more than meets the eye. Alcohol in moderation may actually serve as a better choice.

One study conducted at the Brigham and Women's Hospital in Boston, Massachusetts shows more weight loss by women consuming moderate levels of alcohol versus those drinking other standard juices. However, this is the result when a choice has been made to drink calories, the lesser of two evils.

A quick glance at the components of various drinks may explain the results.

Beverage	Calories	Carbs (g)	Fat (g)
Alcoholic			
Beer (regular)	146	13.13	0
Beer (lite)	99	4.6	0
All Distilled Spirits (rum, vodka, whiskey, gin, tequila, bourbon, etc.)	97	0	0
Wine (red)	125	3.5	0
Wine (white)	120	3.5	0

Non-Alcoholic			
Apple juice (unsweetened)	117	28.96	0.273
Apricot juice	140	36.11	0.226
Carbonated cola	155	39.77	0
Grape juice (unsweetened)	155	37.84	0.202
Grapefruit juice (unsweetened)	94	22.13	0.247
Lemonade	131	34.05	0.149
Milk (2% fat)	122	11.41	4.807
Orange juice (unsweetened)	112	26.84	0.149
Prune juice	182	44.67	0.077
Tangerine juice (unsweetened)	125	29.88	0.098
Tomato juice	41	10.3	0.122

Drinking alcohol during a meal

Normally, after you have eaten a meal, the body will metabolize the food just consumed. Then, that food will be burned for energy. Ultimately, the calories from the food will either be burned off or stored as fat. When alcohol is consumed, however, this process is altered due to the way the body handles alcohol once it is ingested.

The body has a natural process for eliminating alcohol when drinking a significant amount of alcohol before a meal or at the beginning of a meal. The body will have to adjust to processing both the alcohol and food. Processing alcohol is a responsibility of the liver, which produces the enzymes necessary for such a task. This process begins quickly because alcohol is not stored in the body like food. Thus, alcohol must be oxidized and quickly passed during the metabolizing process.

While the gastrointestinal tract is responding to absorb and release alcohol, it does not simultaneously change itself to respond to food that will subsequently be digested. Therefore, food that might normally serve as a source for nutrition may not be efficiently received as such by the body.

The importance of this alcohol induced metabolizing process does not seem to have universal agreement. Some argue that alcohol may prevent the body from processing certain foods, it may allow for weight loss because bad foods would not be processed.

Others contend that once alcohol reaches the stomach and starts being absorbed into the blood stream, all calorie burning comes to a halt. This argument offers that the body perceives alcohol to be a toxin and slows the digestive process to rid itself of that toxin. So, what is not passed through will eventually be stored as fat, making it important not to consume fatty foods with alcohol.

Wherever the truth exists, no one seriously recommends heavily drinking alcohol each day as part of a weight loss or exercise plan. Fortunately, there is a way that you can still drink alcohol and avoid adding on extra pounds. You just need to know when and how to drink alcohol when dieting. The basic rule of course is to drink in moderation (one standard drink for women and two for men). This ensures that the alcohol does not severely interfere with your body's metabolism and guards against inebriation.

The best time of day

The time of day when you sip your favorite wine or beer matters a lot in determining the success of your weight loss program.

In the morning, prior to exercise, your metabolism is still lagging from the dormancy of the night's rest and *breaking* from the overnight *fast*, (i.e. *breakfast*). If you drink alcohol first thing in the morning, you are making your metabolism even slower because of how alcohol will impact your system. Throughout the day, you would experience low metabolism, which would prevent your body from burning as many calories as you may desire. There would also be a dehydrating effect.

In the afternoon and evening, your body is at its peak in terms of metabolism and cognition. A glass of wine will be absorbed more quickly and the body will return to burning calories within a short time. In addition, your brain functioning will not be as affected in the afternoon. So, you can still proceed properly after an afternoon drink. If you are working, however, you may want to reserve the alcohol for late afternoon/early evening after work.

If it is too close to your bedtime, do not drink any alcohol. You may think that it will help you sleep easier, but in the morning you will not feel rested at all. At first, the alcohol will help you get into the deep sleep the body needs for restoration and repair. After a few hours, however, as it wears off, you may wake up and going back to sleep becomes problematic. Also, there may be the need for multiple bathroom trips which will interrupt your sleeping. The result is that in the morning, you will feel tired and exhausted instead of rested.

Moderation is key

Calories from alcoholic drinks can very easily add up and cause considerable weight gain. If you are on a weight loss program, moderating your alcohol intake will help you stay on track. Alcohol intake may reduce energy levels that are necessary for the next work out.

It is possible for alcohol to have impairing affects, even if not consumed in excessive amounts. So, to make sure that your alcohol intake does not negatively impact your health, be mindful of what you have been drinking. Obviously, do not drink and drive. What is the point of looking good and losing weight if you are severely injured or injure someone else because of alcohol?

Conclusion

Now it is up to you. What will you do to make the best schedule for your lifestyle? How and when will you implement what you now know? It is up to you.

Ideas to consider

Breakfast

"A Bigger Breakfast is Better." As the saying goes, "Eat breakfast like a king, lunch like a prince, and dinner like a pauper."

When fruit is consumed on an empty stomach for breakfast, there is time for fiber to create a feeling of being full at the beginning of the day. This will also help in may also assist in adding natural sugars at the beginning of the day. Just beware of the Glycemic Index. Fruits such as pears and apples tend to slow down the release of glucose into your bloodstream. This ultimately stabilizes your blood sugar level.

If you choose to eat carbs for breakfast, eating good complex carbohydrates in the morning will provide your body with energy to set you on the right path for the whole day.

Lunch

White meat such as chicken and fish are ideal for lunch, as they are not as heavy as red meat. Eating protein at lunch allows time to burn off the heaviness of meat and help to build muscle. It will also help to fight snacking temptations that often bring us down later in the afternoon. Protein will be slowly released or stay in the stomach for some time.

Dinner

For those who enjoy having a full-size dinner, but are not able to burn off all the calories burned, a plate full of vegetables may be a great option. Because vegetables are naturally low in calories, vegetables as the primary food at dinner allows for satisfaction without weight gain.

The most beneficial way to eat vegetables is raw. Beware, the most popular salad dressings can cause a major setback in weight loss. The ingredients used in many dressings contain high levels of sugars and calories

No Skipping Meals

Do not skip meals for your diet unless you are working to become a sumo wrestler! Remember sumo wrestlers trying to gain weight do the following:

1. NEVER eat breakfast

2. ONLY eat 1-2 meals a day

3. Sleep after eating

4. Drink large amounts of beer

There should be at least 2-3 hours between bedtime and the last meal of the day. Eating too close to sleeping at night has been associated with a variety of problems such as strokes, insomnia, sleep apnea, acid reflux, and weight gain.

Exercise

If you plan on burning fat fast, capitalize on morning exercise on an empty stomach.

If you want to build your muscles, avoid exercising in the morning and do it in the afternoon or in the evening.

If you have a job that allows for a regularly scheduled lunch, your lunch break could be a good time to hit a nearby gym before heading back to the office. This is particularly true if you find yourself working late nights that make it difficult to get up early in the morning.

If you are crunched for time at home and simply want to get complete some level activity, consider walking during lunch or after work before going home.

Caffeine

While caffeine at an early point of the day will aid in providing greater alertness, the effects may be dulled because of the natural addition of cortisol that peaks (on average) between 8:00 and 9:00 AM. The hours of 9:30 -11:30 a.m. provide for increased and lasting stimulation when considered with releases of cortisol. Another round of caffeine after lunch, between 1:30 and 3:30 p.m., may also provide for effective results that last throughout the day.

Beware of caffeine too late in the day, though. Drinking coffee after 5pm, however, can cause restlessness or trouble falling asleep.

Fluids

Water: A 12 week study by the American Chemical Society in Boston revealed that those who consumed two eight ounce glasses of water before a meals lost an average of 5 pounds more than those who did not.

Consuming water shortly after awakening may be beneficial for overall health because sleep is our longest period without food or liquid. Therefore, it is important to replenish our bodies when we awaken.

Tea: Green tea is an excellent source of caffeine. It will even help you lose weight if consumed often enough.

Coffee: Personal expressions of coffee creativity may actually serve as sources of extra calories that may contradict and inhibit the progress being made to lose weight.

Alcohol: Beware ***alcohol***'s liquid calories and exercising suppressing affects.

You have the knowledge. Now, turn it into power for your health.

Appendix

Glycemic Index/ Load Chart

FOOD	GI (glucose = 100)	Serv. size (grams)	GL per serving
BAKERY PRODUCTS AND BREADS			
Banana cake, made with sugar	47	60	14
Banana cake, made without sugar	55	60	12
Sponge cake, plain	46	63	17
Vanilla cake made from packet mix with vanilla frosting (Betty Crocker)	42	111	24
Apple, made with sugar	44	60	13
Apple, made without sugar	48	60	9
Waffles, Aunt Jemima (Quaker Oats)	76	35	10
Bagel, white, frozen	72	70	25
Baguette, white, plain	95	30	15
Coarse barley bread, 75-80% kernels, average	34	30	7

Hamburger bun	61	30	9
Kaiser roll	73	30	12
Pumpernickel bread	56	30	7
50% cracked wheat kernel bread	58	30	12
White wheat flour bread	71	30	10
Wonder™ bread, average	73	30	10
Whole wheat bread, average	71	30	9
100% Whole Grain™ bread (Natural Ovens)	51	30	7
Pita bread, white	68	30	10
Corn tortilla	52	50	12
Wheat tortilla	30	50	8
BEVERAGES			
Coca Cola®, average	63	250 mL	16
Fanta®, orange soft drink	68	250 mL	23
Lucozade®, original (sparkling glucose drink)	95±10	250 mL	40

Apple juice, unsweetened, average	44	250 mL	30
Cranberry juice cocktail (Ocean Spray®)	68	250 mL	24
Gatorade	78	250 mL	12
Orange juice, unsweetened	50	250 mL	12
Tomato juice, canned	38	250 mL	4
BREAKFAST CEREALS AND RELATED PRODUCTS			
All-Bran™, average	55	30	12
Coco Pops™, average	77	30	20
Cornflakes™, average	93	30	23
Cream of Wheat™ (Nabisco)	66	250	17
Cream of Wheat™, Instant (Nabisco)	74	250	22
Grapenuts™, average	75	30	16
Muesli, average	66	30	16
Oatmeal, average	55	250	13

Instant oatmeal, average	83	250	30
Puffed wheat, average	80	30	17
Raisin Bran™ (Kellogg's)	61	30	12
Special K™ (Kellogg's)	69	30	14
GRAINS			
Pearled barley, average	28	150	12
Sweet corn on the cob, average	60	150	20
Couscous, average	65	150	9
Quinoa	53	150	13
White rice, average	89	150	43
Quick cooking white basmati	67	150	28
Brown rice, average	50	150	16
Converted, white rice (Uncle Ben's®)	38	150	14
Whole wheat kernels, average	30	50	11
Bulgur, average	48	150	12

COOKIES AND CRACKERS			
Graham crackers	74	25	14
Vanilla wafers	77	25	14
Shortbread	64	25	10
Rice cakes, average	82	25	17
Rye crisps, average	64	25	11
Soda crackers	74	25	12
DAIRY PRODUCTS AND ALTERNATIVES			
Ice cream, regular	57	50	6
Ice cream, premium	38	50	3
Milk, full fat	41	250mL	5
Milk, skim	32	250 mL	4
Reduced-fat yogurt with fruit, average	33	200	11

FRUITS			
Apple, average	39	120	6
Banana, ripe	62	120	16
Dates, dried	42	60	18
Grapefruit	25	120	3
Grapes, average	59	120	11
Orange, average	40	120	4
Peach, average	42	120	5
Peach, canned in light syrup	40	120	5
Pear, average	38	120	4
Pear, canned in pear juice	43	120	5
Prunes, pitted	29	60	10
Raisins	64	60	28
Watermelon	72	120	4
BEANS AND NUTS			
Baked beans, average	40	150	6
Blackeye peas, average	33	150	10

Black beans	30	150	7
Chickpeas, average	10	150	3
Chickpeas, canned in brine	38	150	9
Navy beans, average	31	150	9
Kidney beans, average	29	150	7
Lentils, average	29	150	5
Soy beans, average	15	150	1
Cashews, salted	27	50	3
Peanuts, average	7	50	0
PASTA and NOODLES			
Fettucini, average	32	180	15
Macaroni, average	47	180	23
Macaroni and Cheese (Kraft)	64	180	32
Spaghetti, white, boiled, average	46	180	22
Spaghetti, white, boiled 20 min, average	58	180	26
Spaghetti, wholemeal,	42	180	17

boiled, average			
SNACK FOODS			
Corn chips, plain, salted, average	42	50	11
Fruit Roll-Ups®	99	30	24
M & M's®, peanut	33	30	6
Microwave popcorn, plain, average	55	20	6
Potato chips, average	51	50	12
Pretzels, oven-baked	83	30	16
Snickers Bar®	51	60	18
VEGETABLES			
Green peas, average	51	80	4
Carrots, average	35	80	2
Parsnips	52	80	4
Baked russet potato, average	111	150	33
Boiled white potato, average	82	150	21
Instant mashed potato, average	87	150	17

Sweet potato, average	70	150	22
Yam, average	54	150	20
MISCELLANEOUS			
Hummus (chickpea salad dip)	6	30	0
Chicken nuggets, frozen, reheated in microwave oven 5 min	46	100	7
Pizza, plain baked dough, served with parmesan cheese and tomato sauce	80	100	22
Pizza, Super Supreme (Pizza Hut)	36	100	9
Honey, average	61	25	12

Vince Rozier

Vegetable Nutrition Chart

Food	Serv. Size	Total Fiber (g)	Soluble Fiber (g)	Insoluble Fiber (g)
VEGETABLES/LEGUMES				
Artichoke	1 globe	6.5	4.7	1.8
Asparagus	½ cup	1.8	0.7	1.1
Beans				
chick	½ cup	6.2	1.3	4.9
green/string canned	½ cup	1.3	0.5	0.8
kidney	½ cup	5.8	2.9	2.9
lima	½ cup	6.1	2.6	3.6
navy	½ cup	5.8	2.2	3.6
northern	½ cup	5.6	1.4	4.2
pinto	½ cup	7.4	1.9	5.5
soybeans	½ cup	5.1	2.3	2.8
white	½ cup	5.5	1.4	4.1
Beets	½ cup	1.5	0.7	0.8
Bok Choy	½ cup	1.4	0.5	0.9

Broccoli	½ cup	1.4	1.2	1.2
Brussel Sprouts	½ cup	3.3	2	1.3
Cabbage, green	½ cup	1.8	0.8	1
Cabbage, red	½ cup	0.8	0.3	0.5
Carrots	½ cup	2.6	1.1	1.5
Cauliflower, raw	½ cup	2	0.6	1.4
Celery, raw	½ cup	1	0.4	0.7
Collard greens	½ cup	1.3	1.1	0.2
Corn	½ cup	2	0.3	1.7
Cucumber	½ cup	0.4	0.1	0.4
Eggplant	½ cup	1.2	0.3	0.9
Green Peas	½ cup	4.4	1.3	3.1
Jicama, raw	½ cup	3.2	1.7	1.5
Lettuce, iceberg, raw	½ cup	0.4	0.1	0.3
Onion, raw	½ cup	1.4	0.9	0.6
Peas, cooked	½ cup	4.3	1.2	3.1
Peppers, green/red	½ cup	1.3	0.5	0.8
Potato, baked w/skin	1 med	4	1	3

Potato, mashed	½ cup	1.6	0.9	0.7
Potato, sweet	½ cup	3.8	1.4	2.4
Pumpkin, mashed	½ cup	3.6	0.5	3.1
Spinach	½ cup	2.7	0.5	2.2
Spinach, raw	1 cup	0.4	0.1	0.3
Squash, acorn, baked	½ cup	4	2.3	1.7
Tofu	½ cup	1.4	0.9	0.6
Tomato, raw	½ cup	0.9	0	0.9
Water chestnuts	½ cup	1.2	0.9	1.3
Zucchini	½ cup	1.2	0.5	0.7
FRUITS				
Apple, with skin	1 med	3	0.5	2.5
Banana	1 med	2	0.5	1.5
Blackberries	½ cup	3.8	3.1	0.7
Blueberries	½ cup	1.9	0.2	1.7
Cherries	½ cup	1.7	0.5	1.2
Figs, dried	3	4.6	2	2.6
Grapefruit	Med, ½	1.5	1.2	0.3

Grapes	½ cup	0.8	0.3	0.5
Kiwi	1 large	3.1	0.7	2.4
Mango	1 med	3.7	1.5	2.2
Melon	Med, 1/5	0.7	0.2	0.5
Orange	1 med	2	0.5	1.5
Peach	1 med	3.2	1.3	1.9
Pear, with skin	1 med	4.5	0.5	4
Pineapple	½ cup	1	0.1	0.9
Plum	1 large	1.7	0.9	0.8
Prunes	3 med	1.9	1	0.9
Raisins	¼ cup	1.5	0.4	1.1
Raspberries	½ cup	4.2	0.4	3.8
Strawberries	½ cup	1	0	1
GRAINS				
Bagel, wheat	1	3.1	0.9	2.2
Bagel, white	1	1.6	0.6	1
Barley, cooked	½ cup	4.2	0.9	3.3
Bread				
English muffin	1	2	0.5	1.5

french	1 slice	0.8	0.5	0.3
rye	1 slice	1.8	0.8	0.8
white	1 slice	0.6	0.3	0.3
wheat	1 slice	2.5	0.5	2
Cereal				
Cheerios®	1 cup	2.6	1.2	1.4
Corn Flakes®	1 cup	0.7	0	0.7
Fiber One®	½ cup	14	1	13
Kashi® Shredded Wheat	1 cup	6	1	5
Raisin Bran	1 cup	8.4	1.2	7.2
Oatmeal, instant	¾ cup	3	1	2
Couscous, cooked	½ cup	1.3	0.3	1
Millet, cooked	½ cup	3.3	0.6	2.7
Pita, white	7"	1.3	0.7	0.6
Pita, wheat	7"	4.4	0.7	3.7
Rice				
brown, cooked	½ cup	1.7	0.1	1.6
white, cooked	½ cup	0.2	0	0.2
wild, cooked	½ cup	1.5	0.2	1.3
Spaghetti, cooked	1 cup	2	0.5	1.5

Tortilla	6"	1.3	0.2	1.1
OTHER/ SNACKS				
Corn chips	1 cup	1.2	0	1.2
Crackers				
graham	2" square	0.3	0.2	0.1
Ritz®	1 oz	0.5	0.3	0.2
saltine	1oz	1.2	0.4	0.8
Triscuits®	1 oz	0.5	0.2	0.3
Wheat Thins®	1 oz	1.2	0.3	0.9
Peanut butter, chunky	2 Tbl	1.5	0	1.5
Popcorn	1 cup	1	0	1
Potato chips	1 oz	1.4	0.8	0.6
Pretzels	1 oz	1.1	0.3	0.8

Fiber and Protein Content in Spices

Description	Protein (g) Per 100 g	Fiber, total dietary (g) Per 100 g	Carbs, by difference (g) Per 100 g
Spices, anise seed	17.6	14.6	50.02
Spices, basil, dried	22.98	37.7	47.75
Spices, caraway seed	19.77	38	49.9
Spices, cardamom	10.76	28	68.47
Spices, celery seed	18.07	11.8	41.35
Spices, chervil, dried	23.2	11.3	49.1
Spices, chili powder	13.46	34.8	49.7
Spices, coriander leaf, dried	21.93	10.4	52.1
Spices, coriander seed	12.37	41.9	54.99
Spices, cumin seed	17.81	10.5	44.24
Spices, curry powder	14.29	53.2	55.83

Spices, dill seed	15.98	21.1	55.17
Spices, dill weed, dried	19.96	13.6	55.82
Spices, fennel seed	15.8	39.8	52.29
Spices, fenugreek seed	23	24.6	58.35
Spices, marjoram, dried	12.66	40.3	60.56
Spices, mustard seed, ground	26.08	12.2	28.09
Spices, paprika	14.14	34.9	53.99
Spices, parsley, dried	26.63	26.7	50.64
Spices, pepper, black	10.39	25.3	63.95
Spices, pepper, red or cayenne	12.01	27.2	56.63
Spices, pepper, white	10.4	26.2	68.61
Spices, poppy seed	17.99	19.5	28.13
Spices, sage, ground	10.63	40.3	60.73

Fiber and Protein Content in Snacks

Description	Protein (g) Per 100 g	Fiber, total dietary (g) Per 100 g	Carbs, by difference (g) Per 100 g
Baking chocolate, unsweetened, squares	12.9	16.6	29.84
Beverages, KELLOGG'S SPECIAL K20, protein water mix	35.2	37.5	58.4
Beverages, UNILEVER, SLIMFAST Shake Mix, high protein, powder, 3-2-1 Plan	27.87	18.2	47.48
Cocoa, dry powder, unsweetened, processed with alkali	18.1	29.8	58.3
Dairy drink mix, chocolate, reduced calorie, with low-calorie sweeteners, powder	25	9.4	51.4
Formulated bar, MARS SNACKFOOD US, SNICKERS Marathon Double Chocolate Nut Bar	22.35	10.5	52.47

Formulated bar, MARS SNACKFOOD US, SNICKERS Marathon Honey Nut Oat Bar	22.5	11	54.3
Formulated bar, MARS SNACKFOOD US, SNICKERS MARATHON Protein Performance Bar, Caramel Nut Rush	25	12.5	50.5
Granola bar, KASHI TLC Bar, chewy, mixed flavors	18.57	11.4	53.26
Granola bar, KASHI TLC Bar, crunchy, mixed flavors	15	10	62.78
KASHI, H2H Woven Wheat Cracker, Original	10.6	12.2	73.4
KASHI, H2H Woven Wheat Cracker, Roasted Garlic	10.5	12.2	73.2
KASHI, Pilaf, 7 Whole Grain	13.81	12.3	71
KASHI, TLC, Pita Crisps, Sea Salt	10.5	14.7	72.4

KASHI, TLC, Pita Crisps, Zesty Salsa	11	15.3	71.6
KASHI, TLC, Toasted Asiago Crackers	12.7	9.6	66.4
KELLOGG'S, BEANATURAL, Original 3-Bean Chips	22.9	14.2	46.5
MORNINGSTAR FARMS Mediterranean Chickpea, frozen, unprepared	15.5	10.1	19.8
Oriental mix, rice-based	17.31	13.2	51.62
Popcorn, microwave, low fat	12.6	14.2	72
Popcorn, microwave, low fat and sodium	12.6	14.2	73.39
Popcorn, unpopped kernels	10.87	12.7	74
Rice bran, crude	13.35	21	49.69

Fiber and Protein Content in Cereals and Breads

Description	Protein (g) Per 100 g	Fiber, total dietary (g)Per 100 g	Carbs, (g) Per 100 g
Amaranth flakes	15.54	9.5	71.15
GENERAL MILLS, CHEERIOS	12.09	9.4	73.23
KASHI GO LEAN CRUNCH!, Honey Almond Flax	16.9	15.2	66.9
KASHI GOLEAN	26.1	19.6	58
KASHI GOLEAN CRISP Cinnamon Crumble	19.8	17.6	66.1
KASHI GOLEAN CRISP Toasted Berry Crumble	18.1	17.4	68.7
KASHI GOLEAN CRUNCH!	16.6	15.1	73
KASHI Granola, Summer Berry cereal	11.5	13.2	72.4
NATURE'S PATH, OPTIMUM	14.55	18.2	73.37
NATURE'S PATH, OPTIMUM SLIM	16.36	20	69.09
QUAKER, 100% Natural Granola, Oats, Wheat and Honey	10.55	10.2	73.65
SUN COUNTRY,	26.55	10.2	58.11

KRETSCHMER Honey Crunch Wheat Germ			
SUN COUNTRY, KRETSCHMER Toasted Wheat Bran	17.56	41.3	59.51
SUN COUNTRY, KRETSCHMER Wheat Germ, Regular	31.43	11.9	49.38
UNCLE SAM CEREAL	15.98	20.3	65.78
wheat germ, toasted, plain	29.1	15.1	49.6
KASHI GO LEAN Hot Cereal, Creamy TRULY VANILLA, dry	22	19.3	61
KASHI GO LEAN Hot Cereal, Hearty Honey & Cinnamon, dry	19.3	13.2	67
Oats, instant, fortified, plain, dry	11.92	10	69.52
Oats, regular and quick, not fortified, dry	13.15	10.1	67.7
QUAKER, Instant Oatmeal Organic, Regular	16	9.8	67
QUAKER, Instant Oatmeal, Apple and Cinnamon, reduced sugar	10.29	9.7	72.17
QUAKER, Oat Bran,	17.03	14.3	62.94

QUAKER/MOTHER'S Oat Bran, dry			
QUAKER, QUAKER MultiGrain Oatmeal, dry	11.3	12	73.44
QUAKER, Quick Oats with Iron, Dry	13.7	9.4	68.18
QUAKER, Quick Oats, Dry	13.7	9.4	68.18
Bread, reduced-calorie, wheat	13.32	11.1	42.47
Bread, wheat, white wheat	10.66	9.2	43.91
Bread, whole-wheat, commercially prepared, toasted	16.27	9.2	51.16
Buckwheat	13.25	10	71.5
Buckwheat flour, whole-groat	12.62	10	70.59
Chickpea flour (besan)	22.39	10.8	57.82
Wheat bran, crude	15.55	42.8	64.51
Wheat germ, crude	23.15	13.2	51.8
Wheat, hard red spring	15.4	12.2	68.03
Wheat, hard red winter	12.61	12.2	71.18
Wheat, KAMUT khorasan, uncooked	14.54	11.1	70.58
Barley, hulled	12.48	17.3	73.48
Crackers, whole-wheat	10.58	10.3	69.55

References

Appel, L. J., Sacks, F. M., Carey, V. J., Obarzanek, E., Swain, J. F., Miller, E. R., . . . Bishop, L. M. (2005, November 16). Effects of Protein, Monounsaturated Fat, and Carbohydrate Intake on Blood Pressure and Serum Lipids - Results of the OmniHeart Randomized Trial . *The Journal of the American Medical Association, 294*(19), 2455-2464. doi:10.1001/jama.294.19.2455.

Atkinson, F. S., Foster-Powell, K., & Brand-Miller, J. C. (2008, December). International Tables of Glycemic Index and Glycemic Load Values: 2008. *Diabetes Care, 31* (12), pp. 2281-2283. doi:10.2337/dc08-1239

Baxamusa, B. N. (2013, May 15). *List of Complex Carbohydrates*. Retrieved June 2014, from Buzzle: http://www.buzzle.com/articles/complex-carbohydrates-list.html

Biaggioni, I., & Davis, S. N. (2002 , February). Caffeine: A Cause of Insulin Resistance? *Diabetes Care , 25*(2), 399-400. doi:10.2337/diacare.25.2.399

Brown, C. M., Dulloo, A. G., & Montani, J.-P. (2006, September 1). Water-Induced Thermogenesis Reconsidered: The Effects of Osmolality and Water Temperature on Energy Expenditure after Drinking. *91* (9), 3598-3602 . doi:10.1210/jc.2006-0407

Clinical trial confirms effectiveness of simple appetite control method. (2010, August 23). Retrieved June 2014, from American Chemical Society:

http://www.acs.org/content/acs/en/pressroom/newsrel
eases/2010/august/clinical-trial-confirms-
effectiveness-of-simple-appetite-control-method.html

(2001). *Composition of Foods Raw, Processed, Prepared
(USDA Nutrient Database for Standard Reference -
Release 14)*. Beltsville Human Nutrition Research
Center, U.S. Department of Agriculture. USDA
Nutrient Data Laboratory. Retrieved June 2014, from
https://www.ars.usda.gov/SP2UserFiles/Place/12354
500/Data/SR14/sr14_doc.pdf

Davies, M. J., Baer, D. J., Judd, J. T., Brown, E. D., Campbell,
W. S., & Taylor, P. R. (2002, May 15). Effects of
Moderate Alcohol Intake on Fasting Insulin and
Glucose Concentrations and Insulin Sensitivity in
Postmenopausal Women: A Randomized Controlled
Trial. *The Journal of the American Medical
Association, 287*(19), 2559-2562.
doi:10.1001/jama.287.19.2559.

Debono, M., Ghobadi, C., & Ross, R. J. (2009, May).
Modified-Release Hydrocortisone to Provide
Circadian Cortisol Profiles. *The Journal of Clinical
Endocrinology and Metabolism, 94*(5), 1548-1554.
doi:10.1210/jc.2008-2380

(2010). *Dietary Guidelines for Americans*. U.S. Department of
Agriculture and U.S. Department of Health and
Human Services. Washington, D.C. : U.S.
Government Printing Ofice. Retrieved June 2014,
from
http://www.cnpp.usda.gov/Publications/DietaryGuide
lines/2010/PolicyDoc/PolicyDoc.pdf

(2005). *Dietary Reference Intakes for Energy, Carbohydrate,*

Fiber, Fat, Fatty Acids, Cholesterol, Protein, and Amino Acids. INSTITUTE OF MEDICINE OF THE NATIONAL ACADEMIES, The National Academy of Sciences. Washington, D.C.: The National Academies Press. Retrieved June 2014, from http://www.nal.usda.gov/fnic/DRI/DRI_Energy/energy_full_report.pdf

(2005). *Dietary Reference Intakes For Water, Potassium, Sodium, Chloride and Sulfate.* INSTITUTE OF MEDICINE OF THE NATIONAL ACADEMIES, The National Academy of Sciences. Washington, D.C.: The National Academies Press. Retrieved June 2014, from http://www.nal.usda.gov/fnic/DRI/DRI_Water/water_full_report.pdf

Early morning exercise is best for reducing blood pressure and improving sleep. (2011, June 13). Retrieved June 2014, from ASU News - Appalachian State University: http://www.news.appstate.edu/2011/06/13/early-morning-exercise/

Gebhardt, S. E., Haytowitz, D. B., Lemar, L. E., Howe, J. C., Exler, J., Cutrufelli, R. L., . . . Holden, J. M. (2004, February 25). *USDA Nutrient Database for Standard Reference, Release No. 16.1.* Retrieved June 2014, from National Agricultural Library-United States Department of Agriculture: http://www.nal.usda.gov/fnic/foodcomp

Halton, T. L., Willett, W. C., Liu, S., Manson, J. E., Albert, C. M., Rexrode, K., & Hu, F. B. (2006, November 9). Low-Carbohydrate-Diet Score and the Risk of Coronary Heart Disease in Women. *The New*

England Journal of Medicine, 355, 1991-2002 . doi:10.1056/NEJMoa055317

Harding, A. (n.d.). *20 Best Foods for Fiber - High-fiber foods.* Retrieved June 2014, from Health: http://www.health.com/health/gallery/0,,20553010,00 .html

Hermann, J. R. (n.d.). *Protein and the Body.* Retrieved June 2014, from Oklahoma Cooperative Extension Service: http://pods.dasnr.okstate.edu/docushare/dsweb/Get/D ocument-2473/T-3163web.pdf

High, Medium and Low GI Foods. (n.d.). Retrieved June 2014, from The GI Diet Guide: http://www.the-gi-diet.org/lowgifoods/

Hill, D. (2013, August 16). *Drinking Cold Water After Eating.* Retrieved June 2014 , from Livestrong.com: http://www.livestrong.com/article/537267-drinking-cold-water-after-eating/

Lemon, P. W. (1995, Jun). Do athletes need more dietary protein and amino acids? *International Journal of Sport Nutrition, 5*, S39-61. Retrieved June 2014, from http://www.ncbi.nlm.nih.gov/pubmed/7550257

Lovalloa, W. R., Farag, N. H., Vincent, A. S., Thomas, T. L., & Wilson, M. F. (2006, March). Cortisol responses to mental stress, exercise, and meals following caffeine intake in men and women. *Pharmacology Biochemistry and Behavior, 83*(3), 441-447. doi:10.1016/j.pbb.2006.03.005

Mozaffarian, D., Hao, T., Rimm, E. B., Willett, W. C., & Hu, F. B. (2011, June 23). Changes in Diet and Lifestyle and Long-Term Weight Gain in Women and Men. *The New England Journal of Medicine, 364*, 2392-2404. doi:10.1056/NEJMoa1014296

Nutrition Information for Raw Fruits, Vegetables, and Fish - Federal Register. (2006, August 17). Retrieved June 2014, from U.S. Food and Drug Administration: http://www.fda.gov/food/ingredientspackaginglabelin g/labelingnutrition/ucm063367.htm

Ophardt, C. E. (2003). *Alcohol Metabolism Effects*. Retrieved June 2014, from Virtual Chembook-Elmhurst College: http://www.elmhurst.edu/~chm/vchembook/642alcoh olmet.html

Pan, A., Sun, Q., Bernstein, A. M., Schulze, M. B., Manson, J. E., Stampfer, M. J., . . . Hu, F. B. (2012, AprIL 9). Red Meat Consumption and Mortality: Results from Two Prospective Cohort Studies. *Archives of Internal Medicine, 172*(7), 555–563. doi:10.1001/archinternmed.2011.2287

Roehrs, T., & Roth, T. (2001). Sleep, sleepiness, sleep disorders and alcohol use and abuse. *Sleep Medicine Reviews, 5*(4), 287–297. doi:10.1053/smrv.2001.0162

Sherrow, G., & Kirk, E. (2010, January 20). *Balancing Blood Sugar: Why is it important?* Retrieved June 2014, from Hearst Seattle Media, LLC: http://blog.seattlepi.com/naturalmedicine/2010/01/20/ balancing-blood-sugar-why-is-it-important/

Stipp, D. (2012, December 18). How Intermittent Fasting Might Help You Live a Longer and Healthier Life. *Scientific American, 308*(1). Retrieved June 2014, from http://www.scientificamerican.com/article/how-intermittent-fasting-might-help-you-live-longer-healthier-life/?page=1

USDA National Nutrient Database for Standard Reference. (2011, December 7). Retrieved June 2014 , from National Agricultural Library-United States Department of Agriculture: http://ndb.nal.usda.gov/

Van Proeyen, K., Szlufcik, K., Nielens, H., Pelgrim, K., Deldicque, L., Hesselink, M., . . . Hespel, P. (2010 , November 1). Training in the fasted state improves glucose tolerance during fat-rich diet. *The Journal of Physiology, 588*(21), 4289-302. doi:10.1113/jphysiol.2010.196493

Wing, R. R., & Phelan, S. (2005, July). Long-term weight loss maintenance1,2,3,4. *The American Journal of Clinical Nutrition, 82*(1), July . Retrieved from http://ajcn.nutrition.org/content/82/1/222S.full.pdf+html

Wong, S., Jamous, A., O'Driscoll, J., Sekhar, R., Weldon, M., Yau, C. Y., . . . Forbes, A. (2014, February). A Lactobacillus casei Shirota probiotic drink reduces antibiotic-associated diarrhoea in patients with spinal cord injuries: a randomised controlled trial. *British Journal of Nutrition, 111* (04), 672-678. doi:10.1017/S0007114513002973

Wyatt, N. (2014, March 12). *Debunking water myths: weight loss, calorie burn and more*. Retrieved June 2014, from UAB News-The University of Alabama at Birmingham: http://www.uab.edu/news/youcanuse/item/4350-debunking-water-myths-weight-loss-calorie-burn-

and-more

Zelman, K. M. (2011, March 22). *Fiber: How Much Do You Need? Tips and ideas to get more fiber in your diet.* Retrieved June 2014 , from WebMD: http://www.webmd.com/food-recipes/features/fiber-how-much-do-you-need

Vince Rozier